T0367141

Systematic Psychiatric Evaluation

Systematic Psychiatric Evaluation

A Step-by-Step Guide to Applying
The Perspectives of Psychiatry

Margaret S. Chisolm, M.D.
Constantine G. Lyketsos, M.D., M.H.S.

Department of Psychiatry and Behavioral Sciences
The Johns Hopkins University School of Medicine

Foreword by
Paul R. McHugh, M.D., and Phillip R. Slavney, M.D.

The Johns Hopkins University Press
Baltimore

© 2012 The Johns Hopkins University Press
All rights reserved. Published 2012
Printed in the United States of America on acid-free paper
9 8 7 6 5 4 3 2 1

The Johns Hopkins University Press
2715 North Charles Street
Baltimore, Maryland 21218-4363
www.press.jhu.edu

Library of Congress Cataloging-in-Publication Data
Chisolm, Margaret S.
Systematic psychiatric evaluation : a step-by-step guide to applying the perspectives of psychiatry / Margaret S. Chisolm and Constantine G. Lyketsos ; foreword by Paul R. McHugh and Phillip R. Slavney.
p. ; cm.
Includes bibliographical references and index.
ISBN 978-1-4214-0701-2 (hdbk. : alk. paper) —
ISBN 1-4214-0701-9 (hdbk. : alk. paper) —
ISBN 978-1-4214-0702-9 (pbk. : alk. paper) —
ISBN 1-4214-0702-7 (pbk. : alk. paper) —
ISBN 978-1-4214-0869-9 (ebk) — ISBN 1-4214-0869-4 (ebk)
I. Lyketsos, Constantine G. II. Title.
[DNLM: 1. Mental Disorders—diagnosis—Case Reports. 2. Interview, Psychological—Case Reports. WM 141]

616.89′075—dc23   2012002229

Figures from McHugh, PR, Slavney, PR, *The Perspectives of Psychiatry,* Second Edition, © 1998 The Johns Hopkins University Press, are adapted for reproduction with permission of The Johns Hopkins University Press and appear on the pages listed: *from page 52, figure 3:* 7, 63, 82, 97, 117, 127, 140, 160, 176, 196, and 210; *from page 141, figure 8:* 9, 43, 81, 96, 113, 125, 139, 158, 174, 194, and 208; *from page 153, figure 9:* 11, 55, 82, 97, 116, 126, 140, 159, 175, 195, and 209; *from page 259, figure 13:* 12, 36, 80, 95, 111, 125, 138, 157, 174, 193, and 208.

Special discounts are available for bulk purchases of this book. For more information, please contact Special Sales at 410-516-6936 or specialsales@press.jhu.edu.

The Johns Hopkins University Press uses environmentally friendly book materials, including recycled text paper that is composed of at least 30 percent post-consumer waste, whenever possible.

For Richard and Nonnie

Contents

Foreword

Like all teachers, we find great satisfaction in seeing our students apply and advance the ideas they have learned—a satisfaction we felt reading this book. What, though, does the book contribute—to us and, we anticipate, to its readers?

At the simplest level, it consists of case histories—stories of patients with a variety of mental problems who found help from thoughtful psychiatrists in making sense of their difficulties and resolving them. These accounts are interesting purely as stories, but they find their importance in that they go beyond describing the plights of their subjects to illustrate how contemporary psychiatrists must act and think if they are to meet their professional responsibilities.

All the case histories convey two themes tied to coherent clinical practice. First, they display how psychiatrists should garner factual information about a person in the context of his or her life in order to appreciate human mental distress from "within." And second, they express a structure of reasoning about the nature of psychiatric disorders that renders these clinical presentations comprehensible and their optimal treatments distinctive. Know your patient. Think about causes. Make a rational prescription. That's the sequence repeatedly spelled out here.

With this book the authors intend to demonstrate how the concepts we described in *The Perspectives of Psychiatry* work in practice—concepts that we believe are the explicit and traditional ways psychiatrists have for making sense of mental disorders and so helping patients. But why is this book needed now? It is needed because of the problematic state of American psychiatry.

We have previously tried to identify that state. We've said such things as "psychiatry has not come of age," "psychiatry is at a stalemate." By those assertions we meant that in pushing psychiatrists into thinking that their clinical enterprise depended on diagnostic consistency, "*DSM* psychiatry" has, perforce, led them to reflect less and less about what underlies their patients' presentations.

A manual that was intended to quiet sectarian debate about matters of nature and cause *until* they could be better resolved has deprived psychiatrists of the very incentive—that sense of ignorance—needed to *provoke* such a resolution. Under *The Diagnostic and Statistical Manual of Mental Disorders* (*DSM-III/IV*), psychiatric practice has devolved from a thoughtful professional art to a technical, instrumentalist routine where, with what exists being officially presumed, what is done both diagnostically and therapeutically is mechanical and generic rather than devised, individuated, challenging, and progressive.

From official psychiatry there is little in sight that will alter these facts. Those updating the *DSM* in preparation for its fifth edition remain preoccupied with consistency of labeling—a fundamentally instrumentalist practice that emphasizes more what a diagnosis "does" than what it "reveals." A bureaucratic spirit that subordinates concepts of nature and cause to the presumed practical needs for diagnostic consistency has captured the discipline for over thirty years and has, we believe, suppressed its vitality.

Although psychiatrists with *DSM* tunnel vision no longer bear the buoyant self-assurance of psychoanalysts—with their claim to know the very secrets of human life—they do display a complacent satisfaction in refusing to go beyond the securities of diagnostic consistency given to them by the *DSM* diagnostic categories—a complacency often expressed in discussion-ending statements such as "he meets criteria."

Satisfaction of this sort was never the aim of general medicine. Historically, physicians were eager to advance from their professional acquaintance with medical disorders ("knowing *of*" them, as William James might have said) to grasping more and more of their essential natures ("knowing *about*" them) as expressions of biological life. And so, physicians went from knowing *of* fevers, dropsy, palsies, and the like to knowing *about* bodily responses to infection, the edema of heart failure, infarctions of the brain, and so on.

This progression from naming disorders to conceptualizing what generates them advanced slowly but steadily along with the growing alliance of medicine with biology so that today the medical and biological disciplines are encompassed as aspects of the "Life Sciences." Historical figures such as Harvey, Sydenham, Pasteur, and Koch pioneered this progressive course, and all of us are their beneficiaries.

Given that knowledge of psychiatry is ever a participant's knowledge—coming from, growing with, and always related to the practical experience of serving patients—we are provoked to ask why psychiatrists must remain so impoverished in their grasp of the domain of mental life that they cannot move from knowing *of* examples of its disorders (embodied in the current *DSM*'s atheoretical, criterion-driven diagnostic approach) to knowing *about* them in some causal, generative sense.

We believe that a change in the cast of mind of most psychiatrists is needed for the field to mature. They must see mental disorders anew, not simply as collections of identifiable symptoms and signs but as comprehensible expressions of differentiated biopsychosocial processes—specifically diseases, temperaments, motivations, and life encounters—at work, often in combination, in human mental life. This means a change in the way psychiatrists talk with and study patients as well as how they look at themselves as they think about and assess their opinions.

With *The Perspectives of Psychiatry* we did not offer some new theory to psychiatrists but rather drew attention to causal ideas long implicit within the discipline and in need of re-emphasis at this time and place in the discipline's history: specifically ideas that provide psychiatrists power to "know about" the disorders that they now "know of" by name. *The Perspectives of Psychiatry* strives to offer a view of what psychiatry today ought to become. Readers of our text—even if open to its appeal—have often asked how we use our ideas in the daily practice of psychiatry. What would a diagnostic formulation and therapeutic plan based on these concepts look like? Margaret Chisolm and Constantine Lyketsos have provided just such practical demonstrations with the case histories in this book.

We are indebted to them for illustrating so skillfully how using the concepts of diseases, dimensions, behaviors, and life stories can enrich the care of patients and integrate emerging scientific knowledge about mental life into the daily practice of clinicians. Our satisfaction as teachers of them is more than matched by our gratitude to them for what they have presented here.

Paul R. McHugh, M.D., and Phillip R. Slavney, M.D.

Preface

This book has been in our thoughts for over twenty years. Its development was stimulated by our clinical use of the systematic approach presented by Drs. McHugh and Slavney in *The Perspectives of Psychiatry*. We saw the power of the *Perspectives* approach demonstrated time after time with patients—and our students appreciated its theoretical underpinnings. But they and we recognized the need to distill that book's concepts into an easier-to-digest and easier-to-use format. *Systematic Psychiatric Evaluation* is our attempt to distill the detailed instructions of *The Perspectives of Psychiatry* into a practical "recipe" for trainees.

About *Systematic Psychiatric Evaluation*

We have divided the book into two major parts. The purpose of part 1 is to illustrate key concepts. We begin with an introduction to the systematic and integrative approach to understanding patients as presented in *The Perspectives of Psychiatry*. Chapter 1 serves as an introduction (or review) of the methods presented there. Each subsequent chapter in part 1 uses a case to illuminate the key concepts underlying each of the four perspectives. Part 1 does *not* provide formulations for the cases.

Part 2 consists of nine cases demonstrating how the *Perspectives* approach can effectively be used in practice. Each case presentation is followed by a systematic formulation interweaving each of the perspectives, from which an integrative treatment plan is ultimately developed. We hope that this easy-to-read format will help clinicians learn to use the approach and thereby develop complete and personalized formulations of individual cases.

About the Cases

All of the case presentations (with the exception of the one in chapter 2) are drawn from patients treated by us and a handful of other Hopkins psychiatrists over the years. (As neither of us is a child and adolescent psychiatrist, only adult patient cases are included in this book, although the approach can also be used to evaluate children and adolescents who present with psychiatric signs and symptoms. We anticipate another volume of this case book focused on how to apply the *Perspectives* approach to the mental health problems of children and adolescents.) To prevent the personal identification of patients and families, we synthesized histories from several patients to create the composite cases presented. In addition, we removed or disguised all identifying details by using pseudonyms and altering gender, occupation, location, etc. However, we kept untouched, and therefore real, the essential clinical features of each case. We use schematic figures liberally to illustrate concepts and provide a bulleted summary of key points at the end of each chapter/case.

We discuss the systematic *Perspectives* approach to the history, mental status exam (MSE), and formulation in some detail over the course of the book. Chapter 2 focuses on the essential features of the psychiatric evaluation necessary for the application of the approach. All subsequent presentations in this book differ in several ways from the case in chapter 2. First, the cases are based on evaluations of actual patients. Second, for readability, each case is presented in an abridged, dialogue format. Thus, no single case represents a complete rendering of any particular patient's history as originally obtained. We hope, however, that the reader will finish the book with a full appreciation of a comprehensive history, MSE, and formulation. Appendix A is a "bedside" version of the psychiatric evaluation format, including the MSE, used at Johns Hopkins. Appendix B is a "bedside" version of the MSE used at Hopkins and a discussion of its components and application.

Acknowledgments

We are grateful to the many Johns Hopkins medical students and psychiatry residents who worked closely with us from 2006 to 2012. In talking about the book's ideas and reading drafts of the text they helped us bring this case book to fruition. We are especially grateful to those students and residents who helped us with the book's research and case presentations. Most specifically, we thank those who put in many hours to help develop this volume: Allan Andersen, Charles Arthur, Aaron Bobb, Crystal Clark, Sean Heffernan, Meghann Hennelly, Amy Huberman, Geneva Massiello, Megan Mrozckowski, Teresa O'Herron, Matthew Peters, Joanna Pearson, Anne Ruble, Lee Spencer, Sarah Tighe, and Elizabeth Winters. We are also immensely grateful to the many patients whom we have had the privilege to treat and who have taught us so much about taking care of patients with psychiatric conditions.

The faculty and staff of the Johns Hopkins Department of Psychiatry and Behavioral Sciences and other departments and schools of medicine, as well as staff from the Johns Hopkins Bayview Medical Center, contributed to the book both by providing general comments and through specific research or technical support. Specifically, we thank: Kimberly Allan, Catherine DeAngelis, James Harris, Adam Kaplin, Dean MacKinnon, Lawrence Mayer, Donna Mennitto, Karin Neufeld, Joan Nicaise, Peter Rabins, Vani Rao, Cheri Smith, Constance Tawney, and Barbara Verrier.

We give special thanks to our family and friends for their various forms of support for the project. Thank you, Richard and Jasper Chisolm; Nonnie, Theo, and Daphne Lyketsos; Tim Ford, Nancy Hackerman, and Ellen Lupton.

We also want to recognize the interest and enthusiasm of Jacqueline

Wehmueller, our editor at the Johns Hopkins University Press, whose insights and guidance turned our twenty-year dream into a readable reality.

Finally, this book would not have been possible without the vision of Paul McHugh and Phillip Slavney, our personal teachers and role models, who originally articulated the approach in their seminal textbook *The Perspectives of Psychiatry* and contributed immensely to this companion case book. We are forever grateful for the intelligence and kindness that informs their mentorship.

PART I

The Concepts
behind the Approach

CHAPTER ONE

An Introduction

There are these two young fish swimming along and they
happen to meet an older fish swimming the other way, who nods
at them and says, "Morning, boys. How's the water?" And the
two young fish swim on for a bit and then eventually one of them
looks over at the other and goes, "What the hell is water?"

—from *This Is Water,* by David Foster Wallace

Each of us has a mind that is constantly producing an array of thoughts, feelings, and behaviors. Like the water in which David Foster Wallace's young fish swim, our omnipresent mental life often exists on the fringe of our awareness. And when the mind goes awry, its problems can be difficult to recognize. It is usually only when psychiatric conditions reach a certain severity that they come to the attention of a doctor (and then most likely a primary care physician, not a psychiatrist).[1, 2]

Psychiatrists are experts in the evaluation and treatment of patients with disordered thoughts, feelings, and behavior. The American Psychiatric Association's *Diagnostic and Statistical Manual of Mental Disorders* (from *DSM-III* through *DSM-V*) and George Engel's biopsychosocial model[3] provide the basis for psychiatry's current approach to these conditions. The *DSM*'s creation of distinct categories of psychiatric conditions, based on the signs and symptoms with which patients present, allowed researchers to study reliably similar groups of patients and led to advancements in prognosis and treatment. The *DSM* also provides a vernacular that may be used by any clinician, including nonpsychiatrists and nonphysicians, to describe a collection of symptoms displayed by a patient and "assign" a diagnosis based on what is observed. The biopsychosocial

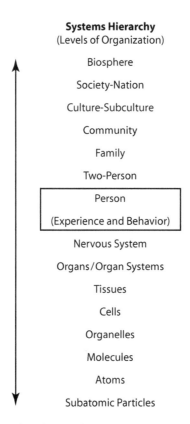

Systems Hierarchy
(Levels of Organization)

Biosphere

Society-Nation

Culture-Subculture

Community

Family

Two-Person

Person

(Experience and Behavior)

Nervous System

Organs/Organ Systems

Tissues

Cells

Organelles

Molecules

Atoms

Subatomic Particles

FIGURE 1.1. Engel's hierarchy of natural systems. *Source:* Engel, GL. The clinical application of the biopsychosocial model. *Am J Psychiatry* 13: 535–544, 1980, p. 537. Reprinted with permission from the *American Journal of Psychiatry* (Copyright 1980). American Psychiatric Association.

model reminds clinicians to consider the multiple and complex aspects of an individual—from subatomic particles to the biosphere. It provides the list of ingredients relevant to all medical diagnosis, modified for psychiatry.

Moving beyond the *DSM* and the biopsychosocial model, Paul McHugh and Phillip Slavney freshly articulated a rigorous and comprehensive conceptual framework for understanding patients who present with psychiatric conditions. Their book, *The Perspectives of Psychiatry*,[4] set out four perspectives: disease, dimensional, behavior, and life story. It laid the foundation for a pragmatic approach to patients based on the nature and origin of the psychiatric condition with which they present. *The Perspectives of Psychiatry* assembled the biopsychosocial model's essential ingredients into a systematic approach to patient care. Our book sets down for the first time the detailed sequence of steps embedded in the *Perspectives* conceptual framework.

Although the essence of this book is case presentation and discussion, the fundamentals of the *Perspectives* approach—a systematic and comprehensive psychiatric assessment and a summary of those concepts central to each of the four perspectives—are introduced here. For a complete explication of these concepts and others, the reader is referred to the source text, *The Perspectives of Psychiatry*.[4]

The central tenet of the *Perspectives* is that one single method cannot explain all psychiatric conditions. The *Perspectives* advocates that a clinician consider every psychiatric patient from four points of view, each with a unique way of understanding the emergence of various psychiatric conditions. Only then, from this fuller understanding, can a clinician develop a truly complete and individualized formulation of the case and treatment plan for the patient. Considering each patient presentation in this way is necessary because psychiatric conditions differ in their fundamental natures. Whereas general medical conditions are always understood as diseases (i.e., clinical syndromes produced by pathological processes arising from physical etiologies), psychiatric conditions cannot be understood consistently in the same way. This is because psychiatric conditions can vary significantly in their probable origins. Some, such as dementia, arise like a general medical disorder, from a "broken part"; others, such as grief, demoralization, sociopathy, and voyeurism, seem to originate in other ways. Thus, the single method employed to figure out the origins of a general medical condition (disease reasoning) may be only partially useful, at best, to understanding patients with psychiatric presentations. To fully formulate the case of a patient who presents with psychiatric symptoms, we must expand our modes of explanation. Although researchers are still attempting to elucidate the causal origin of most psychiatric conditions, the *Perspectives* approach provides practical tools that clinicians need now to diagnose and treat patients. By using this approach *with every patient*, a clinician can both know the patient better as a person and make the formulation of the case and treatment of the patient more complete and effective. This approach can be adopted by clinicians working across a wide range of clinical settings.

The Perspectives of Psychiatry is a text whose objective is to introduce "*perspectival*" thinking as a logical way to understand the field of psychiatry. It has formed the basis for teaching psychiatry to a generation of medical students and psychiatrists. Both *The Perspectives of Psychiatry* and our book are less concerned with the differentiation and classification of psychiatric conditions (nosology) than with helping clinicians become aware of how they think about each patient presentation. Using these methods, readers will learn to become better diagnosticians, better prognosticators, better therapists, and better overall clinicians.

A systematic and comprehensive psychiatric assessment is the essential first step of *Perspectives* reasoning and the foundation for all that follows. A more complete description of the *Perspectives* patient assessment is presented in chapter 2. This type of evaluation can take more than one hour, which in a real-world inpatient or outpatient setting may require more than one visit to complete. However, to employ the *Perspectives* approach successfully, the clinician must devote time and attention to a careful and personalized assessment. This more complete understanding of the patient's condition will reap rewards in the form of the most effective and appropriate treatment plan.

McHugh and Slavney use a visual metaphor (viewing a patient presentation from different points of view, or perspectives) to describe the four ways by which we think about a patient whose thoughts, feelings, and behavior have gone awry. As noted, they refer to these as the disease, dimensional, behavior, and life-story perspectives. In the rest of this chapter, we will briefly present the central concepts of each of these perspectives. Each chapter in the rest of part 1 uses a single case to illustrate concepts central to a particular perspective. These chapters are *not* intended to demonstrate how the four perspectives—in sequence—are actually applied and synthesized to understand a patient's psychiatric presentation. Nor are they intended to discuss in any detail how a case is to be formulated and a patient treated. Instead, each presents a relatively uncomplicated case to convey the key features of a single perspective. The full application of the *Perspectives* approach, which brings all four perspectives to bear on the understanding of every case to develop a formulation and treatment plan, will be demonstrated in part 2, where we introduce cases of increasing complexity.

The Disease Perspective

The disease perspective rests on logic familiar to all physicians—disease reasoning. For psychiatry, as for other medical fields, the disease perspective assumes that a patient's presentation consists of a pattern of signs and symptoms that run a particular course, known as a clinical *syndrome*. In disease reasoning, this recognizable clinical *syndrome* emerges from an underlying *pathology* ("broken part") as a result of one or more *etiologies*. For example, a patient may develop fatigue (symptom) with fever (sign). If these are accompanied by cough, chest pain, shortness of breath, and expectoration, the *syndrome* likely originates in pulmonary *pathology* whose *etiology* may be infectious, neoplastic, immunologic, or another process. Similarly, psychiatric conditions presenting as clinical *syndromes* likely emerge from underlying brain *pathology* whose *etiology* may or may not be known. The key features, then, of the disease perspective are clinical *syndrome, pathology,* and *etiology.*

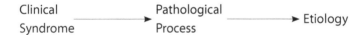

An example of a psychiatric condition that can be best understood from the disease perspective is dementia (a global cognitive decline in the absence of delirium), usually due to loss of brain tissue, which—in turn—can arise from many etiologies (Alzheimer disease and traumatic brain injury being the most common causes in the old and young, respectively). In essence, a disease is something an individual *has.* The driving force is the pathologic process that affects the brain and exerts an effect on a patient's thoughts, feelings, and behavior in life-altering ways. When all three elements of the process (*syndrome, pathology,* and *etiology*) are elucidated for a patient's psychiatric disease, treatments based on a causal link between *etiology,* brain *pathology,* and clinical *syndromes* become possible.

Personality is composed of enduring cognitive and temperament dimensions. The dimensional perspective considers whether a patient's psychiatric condition is arising from aspects of personality that make her vulnerable to developing distress in specific situations. For example, the cognitive dimension of intelligence, usually measured by IQ, develops early in life and stabilizes at an enduring level by early adulthood. Slight decline occurs in adulthood, followed by accelerated decline in late life (even in the absence of dementia). On the other hand, temperament dimensions, typically five, achieve stability by early adulthood and remain stable through the life course.[5] The robust nature of these five dimensions (neuroticism, extraversion, openness, agreeableness, and conscientiousness) has been demonstrated via personality inventories,[5] meta-analyses,[6] and linguistic models.[7] When leveraged successfully, *where* an individual rests on the dimensions of intelligence and temperament can correlate with success in life ("using one's gifts"). (Intelligence, for instance, is a major predictor of educational and occupational attainment.[8, 9]) At the same time, where one rests on these same dimensions can be a source of significant distress. For example, a person of slightly below-average intelligence who grows up in a family of high-achieving parents and siblings might inadvertently be pushed by the family beyond his abilities to the point of distress and maladaptive behavior. Or, a shy, introverted person with an otherwise successful career might falter when put in the position of leading a team, interacting with subordinates, and giving inspirational speeches. In both cases, the person is able to thrive in circumstances suited to his cognition or temperament, but develops psychiatric symptoms when encountering situations that do not fit with who he *is*.

A patient who rests on the extreme of a dimension, whether cognition or temperament, may be vulnerable to psychiatric distress in many circumstances and, thus, exhibit a chronic and pervasive pattern of maladaptive behavior. For example, a patient with an extremely low level of intelligence yet normal temperament may display emotional outbursts when placed in any work environment, consistently lose jobs, and then become distressed about the inability to hold stable employment. Using *DSM* terminology, only patients at the extreme of temperament dimensions are said to have personality disorders. For these individuals an extreme temperament is the primary reason for seeking treatment. In addition, dimensional characteristics can play a role in many psychiatric presentations, even in individuals who do not have personality disorders by *DSM* criteria. Understanding a patient's dimensional characteristics helps the clinician guide the patient in psychotherapy.

The key concepts of the dimensional perspective are *potentials* (where an individual rests on the relevant dimension), *provocations* (the specific circumstance of poor fit for the individual), and *responses* (the feelings and behavior that result from that poor fit).

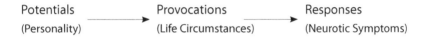

Potentials	Provocations	Responses
(Personality)	(Life Circumstances)	(Neurotic Symptoms)

In this perspective, the patient's psychiatric condition arises from a poor fit between who the person *is* and his circumstances. Treatment initially consists of helping the patient recognize and accept who he is (at times with the aid of psychological testing). As it is usually not possible to change greatly where one rests on dimensions of cognition and temperament, this is followed by guidance to help the patient adapt to who he is by noticing, anticipating, managing, and avoiding (if applicable) circumstances that provoke distress.

The Behavior Perspective

The behavior perspective focuses on what a patient is *doing*. It recognizes that classical and operant conditioning can shape an individual's behavior. What a person does can be affected by what she did yesterday (habit) and by a behavior's rewards and "punishments." These rewards and punishments can be intrinsic, extrinsic, or a combination of the two, producing innate and/or acquired drives. In this perspective, behavior is the central focus. Behavioral choice results from learning, which is based in prior experience (with associated rewards, punishment, and cues) that creates drives. Considering the relevance of this perspective to a particular patient is essentially an exercise in seeing whether the patient's condition can be explained as the result of choice, learning, rewards, punishments, cues, drives, or other forces.

The behavior perspective can be used to explain extraordinary behaviors, such as suicide or homicide. However, it is commonly invoked to explain repetitive maladaptive behaviors involving disruption of everyday innate goal-related activities (e.g., eating, drinking, sexuality) or acquired activities (e.g., substance abuse, gambling). The innately driven activities are governed by fundamental human cycles of strong desire ("hunger"— for food, water, or sex), satiation (after the desire is fulfilled), and latency (when desire for food, water, or sex wanes). These cycles have basic physiologic underpinnings that serve these natural activities. This normal physiology is "hijacked" when a specific innate or acquired behavior gains such salience that an individual chooses to engage in the behavior over and over again to the increasing exclusion of other behaviors. As the cycle continues, the maladaptive behavior becomes so central that relationships and social successes are left behind and the patient becomes isolated and faces recurrent losses. At the same time, by virtue of repetition, the patient's ability *to choose not to engage* in the maladaptive behavior diminishes. Behavioral disorders emerge when an individual becomes stuck in a cycle of repetitively engaging in a behavior to meet a strongly desired goal. The goal might be to have sexual relations with a minor (e.g., pedophilia), to be thin (e.g., anorexia nervosa), or to ingest a substance (e.g., alcohol and drug disorders). Meeting the goal is constantly reinforced by prior experience and is maintained in part by specific rewards (e.g., euphoria), avoidance of punishment (e.g., drug withdrawal), cues, or simply the "comfort" of not changing. In this perspective, normal physiologic underpinnings of everyday behavioral cycles are hijacked, leading to maladaptive behavioral cycles. In some cases, the brains of patients with behavioral disorders *may* be completely normal. A "broken part" in the brain, therefore, is not necessary to explain the problem.

The key concepts behind the behavioral perspective are *choice* (initial choice and late disruption of free choice), *physiological drive* (development of a desire for the maladaptive behavior that is experienced with the same salience as an everyday drive for food, water, or sleep), and *conditioned learning* (maintenance of the behavior by the rules of conditioned learning theory).

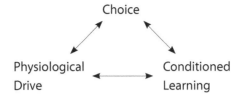

Choice

Physiological Drive ↔ Conditioned Learning

In essence, a behavior is something an individual *does*. Treatment of behavioral disorders consists of applying the rules learned from conditioned learning theory to stop the behavior. This begins with interrupting the maladaptive behavior for a sufficiently long time so the drive is able to gradually extinguish. It is followed by a systematic effort to limit exposure to rewards, cues, or thoughts that may provoke the behavior while putting in place a plan to manage a relapse (typically inevitable in the earliest periods of recovery).

The Life-Story Perspective

Finally, we come to the life-story perspective. Using this perspective, a clinician employs the logic of narrative to help a patient explain the origin of his psychiatric condition in a more adaptive way. Every individual goes through life as an agent with needs, desires, goals, and hopes. When someone *encounters* life circumstances that disrupt these, distress and demoralization may arise (depending on the person and the circumstance). Demoralization is a state of mind in which one has the sense of losing mastery over circumstances.[10] It can be temporary or sustained and does not usually result in a psychiatric presentation. Almost everyone experiences demoralization at some point in life and is usually able to adapt. For those individuals who do present to a clinician for help, the life-story perspective attempts to explain distress in the face of disruption of hopes, goals, dreams, or relationships by everyday circumstances as demoralization.

Grief is an example of a psychiatric phenomenon to which life-story reasoning can be readily applied. Grief is a normal reaction, for example, to the death of a loved one. Almost everyone has experienced grief and can relate to the impact it has on one's life. Loss of a loved one results in predictable outcomes: emotional numbness, followed by disbelief and recurrent memories of the deceased, with "wellings" of sadness and crying. Sleep, appetite, and daily activity might be disrupted. Over time, this state slowly resolves and recedes into the background of the mind, especially when accompanied by the support of others and the resumption of daily activity. Morale is restored and life eventually moves on, although even years later memory of the deceased might trigger a brief "welling" spell. Some individuals seek a clinician's help to deal with the experience of grief.

The life-story perspective emphasizes that a patient's psychiatric presentation, or some aspect of it, arises from an understandable psychological reaction to life's events, often a loss or other challenging circumstance. The essential feature is that a stressful event has occurred that can explain, in a meaningful way, how the patient now feels or behaves. The event interacts with the individual's personality. The reaction is almost always proportionate in content and severity to the stress and is usually consistent with the patient's past reaction to similar events. The clinician can relate as a human being to the patient's experience, but appreciates that different people will have dissimilar reactions to similar circumstances, depending on individual vulnerability. In the life-story perspective, therefore, an individual's psychiatric condition is understood as arising from the *encounter* with a life event that has affected the patient in a way that is understandable to other humans. The conceptual triad of the life-story perspective is like any narrative: *setting, sequence,* and *outcome.*

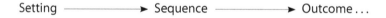

Setting ⟶ Sequence ⟶ Outcome . . .

The clinician must understand what a patient has *encountered* and how it has affected her. Treatment consists of helping the patient organize an interpretation of life events into a narrative that is more effective, active, and optimistic. With this healthier interpretation of the meaning of life events, this narrative, forged collaboratively by the clinician and the patient, helps the patient move forward in life. Notably, this perspective might be used to help the patient adapt to having developed a condition better understood as a disease (e.g., schizophrenia). In that case, the treatment helps the person consider alternative ways of thinking about her life (also known as rescripting) in the presence of a catastrophic illness.

Just as in medicine, where we consider a case as arising from various origins (marked by the mnemonic VITAMIN C: Vascular, Infectious, Toxic, Autoimmune, Metabolic, Idiopathic, Neoplastic, Congenital), in psychiatry the *Perspectives* approach allows us to consider a case as arising from something a patient *has, is, does,* and/or *encounters,* represented by the mnemonic HIDE.

Has
Is
Does
Encounters

A disorder of mental life and behavior doesn't occur in a vacuum but is always embedded in the life of a patient. Recognizing this, it becomes clear that thinking of psychiatric conditions simply as diagnoses is inadequate. Psychiatric conditions arise from and are shaped by an individual's life. In applying the *Perspectives* approach to a patient presenting with psychiatric symptoms, the evaluating clinician must perform more than a check-list assessment, deciding whether the patient meets criteria for *DSM* diagnosis. To understand the origins of a patient's troubles, develop a robust formulation, and prescribe complete treatment using the *Perspectives* approach, the clinician needs to perform an in-depth, *systematic* psychiatric evaluation. That is where everything begins and upon which the entire *Perspectives* approach rests. And it is to the psychiatric evaluation that we now turn.

Summary Points

The points discussed in this chapter are summarized in the figure on the following page.

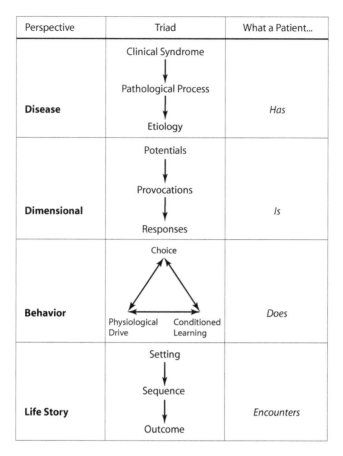

Perspective	Triad	What a Patient...
Disease	Clinical Syndrome ↓ Pathological Process ↓ Etiology	*Has*
Dimensional	Potentials ↓ Provocations ↓ Responses	*Is*
Behavior	Choice △ Physiological Drive — Conditioned Learning	*Does*
Life Story	Setting ↓ Sequence ↓ Outcome	*Encounters*

FIGURE 1.2. The four perspectives of psychiatry. *Source:* Adapted from Rao V, Handel S, Vaishnavi S, Keach S, Robbins B, Spiro J, Ward J, and Berlin F. Psychiatric sequelae of traumatic brain injury: A case report *Am J Psychiatry* 164: 730, 2007. Adapted by Tim Ford and reprinted with permission from the *American Journal of Psychiatry* (Copyright 2007). American Psychiatric Association.

CHAPTER TWO

The Psychiatric Evaluation

Mental disease . . . is, for the most part, dependent upon evidence
which is cognizable by the intellect alone, and upon data which
the senses furnish to us only at second hand. The physician is
compelled to bring to this investigation, not only a knowledge of
those functions which are subservient to the vegetative and animal
life of the individual, but also a clear and analytical conception of
those which collectively constitute mind.

— from Bucknill and Tuke's *Manual of Psychological Medicine*

In this chapter, we present two versions of a single case to illustrate
how a clinician's conception of psychiatric conditions informs the
approach to the psychiatric evaluation and, in turn, the formulation of
the case. The first version represents a typical approach to a psychiatric
history. The second version, of the same case, uses the more comprehensive approach that is fundamental to the *Perspectives*. We present these
two versions not to build a purely logical argument for the superiority of
one method over the other, but to demonstrate that how clinicians think
about psychiatric conditions informs the method of evaluation and influences the understanding of patients and ultimately the outcome of their
treatment.

The Case: Version 1

Informants: The informants for this history included Mr. P and a
friend. Mr. P was lucid only intermittently.

Chief Complaint: Mr. P is a 40-year-old man with a long history of alcohol misuse who was brought to the hospital by his friend because of intoxication.

History of Present Illness: One week prior to admission, en route from Richmond to New York, Mr. P stopped off in Baltimore to visit friends. The friend who brought him to the hospital noted no change in Mr. P's usual routines in the prior week. As was his usual habit when in Baltimore, Mr. P spent most of his time frequenting the city's various bars. On the evening of admission, while drinking in Gunner's Tavern, a fellow patron noted Mr. P to be incoherent and strangely dressed in someone else's clothes. This customer alerted Mr. P's friend, who brought him to the hospital. Mr. P was taking no medications. The review of systems was significant for fever, chills, coughing phlegm, nausea, vomiting, headache, confusion, and dizziness.

Past Medical History: Mr. P has no known drug allergies. During periods of heavy alcohol use and subsequent withdrawal, Mr. P often experiences severe gastrointestinal distress and diarrhea, which he attributes to "the cholera, or spasms quite as bad." He has no known surgical history.

Past Psychiatric History: His friend said that Mr. P becomes depressed when he drinks and often goes to bed for three or four days. He said that Mr. P has had several periods of sobriety, but none lasting more than a few months. Mr. P himself denied ever being depressed during these sober periods and agreed that his mood changes only when he starts drinking. Mr. P described himself as "gravely traumatized" by the death of his mother and subsequent separation from his siblings. Mr. P had few friends growing up, which he attributed to his peers' jealousy of his academic and athletic prowess.

Mr. P said that he was once married, but his wife died some years ago. After her death, while drinking heavily, he had an "abysmal depression." Mr. P then went on to describe fighting a duel over a woman in France, after which a noble Scotswoman visited him daily and nursed him to health. (It was unclear whether this event is true.) Mr. P denied any past psychiatric hospitalizations or other treatment for psychiatric conditions. Mr. P said he never used marijuana, heroin, cocaine, or other drugs, although he said he once tried to end his life. This occurred in the setting of romantic entanglement with two different women, of whom he preferred the younger, married, one. Confused and in an "agony of grief," Mr. P drank half a bottle of laudanum. An unidentified friend induced him to vomit and likely saved his life.

Substance Abuse History: Mr. P became angry when the examiner referred to his drinking. Mr. P said he has tried to cut down on his alcohol intake. He also acknowledged he needed an "eye opener" most mornings.

Family History: Mr. P's father had a history of alcoholism. His mother died at 24 years from an infection; she had no psychiatric history. He had two siblings, one of whom had severe alcoholism and likely died due to a drinking-related illness.

The Case: Version 2

Informants: The informants for this history included Mr. P, a friend, his mother-in-law, and two paternal cousins. Mr. P was lucid only intermittently.

Chief Complaint: Mr. P is a 40-year-old man with a long history of alcohol misuse who was brought to the hospital by his friend because of intoxication.

Family History: Mr. P's father left the family when Mr. P was less than 2 years old, and Mr. P had no further contact with him. His father came from a lower-middle-class family in Baltimore and had abandoned law studies to pursue acting, in which he did poorly by all accounts. Relatives described Mr. P's father as arrogant, quick tempered, and proud; he also struggled with severe alcoholism.

Mr. P's mother died from an "infectious fever" at 24 years old, just shy of Mr. P's third birthday. She was an actress and reportedly gifted singer who led a difficult and strained personal life. She married at age 15, was widowed by age 18, and then married Mr. P's father at 19, only to be left alone again at age 23. Through this, she had no signs or symptoms consistent with psychiatric conditions, including substance abuse.

Mr. P was the middle of three children. His brother (William) was two years older. When their mother died, the children were split up and William was sent to live with relatives in Baltimore. William had a history of alcoholism and died at age 23 from what was likely an alcohol-related illness. Mr. P's sister (Rosalie) is two years younger. She lives in Richmond, Virginia, with a well-to-do family and was described as "slow witted," possibly with intellectual disabilities.

In the extended family, Mr. P's paternal side has a strong history of alcohol abuse and possible depression. His mother's family history is largely unknown. There is no history of suicide in the family.

After his mother's death, Mr. P was taken in by "fans" of his mother. Mr. P's guardian (John) was described by Mr. P to his friends as a "brusque," "hardened," business entrepreneur who gave Mr. P a good education and numerous privileges while growing up; however, their relationship became contentious, largely over the issue of money. John's wife (Frances) was described by Mr. P as "sweet" and "loving." According to the family, Frances has frequent illnesses that her physicians suspect have no physical origin.

Personal History: Mr. P was born in Boston, the product of a full-term, uncomplicated pregnancy, by normal spontaneous vaginal delivery. He was a healthy infant and active child with few, if any, medical problems. His first three years of life were largely itinerant, traveling from city to city with his actor parents. After his mother's death in Richmond, Mr. P was taken in by his guardian family. He lived with this family in Richmond until the age of 9, when they all moved to England for six years so his guardian father could pursue a business venture. After Mr. P's return to the United States, he lived in several cities on the East Coast, including Richmond, Baltimore, Philadelphia, New York, and Boston, but never spent more than two or three years in a single place due to financial constraints.

Mr. P's home life as a child was varied. Separated from his siblings after their mother's death, he moved in with his guardian family. He was treated well by them, but missed his brother. He was never officially adopted by his guardian family, making his status in their household ambiguous (for instance, his foster aunt never accepted Mr. P as part of the family and refused to acknowledge him). As Mr. P grew older, he and his guardian father frequently clashed over monetary issues, with his guardian being alternately generous and stingy. Additionally, his guardian father did not support Mr. P's artistic aspirations.

Mr. P received a strong education. He excelled at languages and English composition and was always at the top of his class. He entered the

University of Virginia at age 16. During his eight months at university, he thrived scholastically, earning top honors at the end of that year. However, he was forced to quit school for financial reasons and, by the time he quit, had accrued a large amount of debt. Mr. P spent a year at West Point during his mid-twenties, and excelled there until he allegedly garnered several infractions deliberately, which led to a court martial and expulsion.

Although he worked for several newspapers and magazines in editorial positions, Mr. P held no job for more than a year. Instead he made money by selling his own writings of poetry, fiction, and literary criticism. This income was frequently insufficient to support him and his family, however, and he has lived most of his adult life in poverty.

Mr. P had no history of physical or sexual abuse.

Mr. P had several romantic relationships in his life. As a teenager, he was engaged to a 15-year-old girl in Richmond but their relationship was thwarted by Mr. P's guardian father, who felt he was too young to marry. At age 23, Mr. P was engaged, but the relationship was tempestuous and ended due to his jealousy and anger over the woman's male friends. At age 26, Mr. P fell in love with and married Virginia, his reportedly 13-year-old first cousin (although the marriage license allegedly states her age as 21). For the rest of Virginia's life, Mr. P lived with her and her mother in a tight-knit family unit. It is unclear whether Mr. P and Virginia's marriage was ever consummated, as he constantly referred to her as his "sister, [his] dearest one." Virginia died twelve years later from tuberculosis, when Mr. P was age 38. After her death, Mr. P became involved with at least four different women. He reported that the woman he loved best was married and thus unavailable to him.

Mr. P does not approve of organized religion and although he identified himself as Christian and said he believes in God, he does not attend church.

Mr. P was never arrested, but he prosecuted a libel suit against a publisher for an article that he believed defamed him.

Past Medical History: Mr. P has no known drug allergies. During periods of heavy alcohol use and subsequent withdrawal, Mr. P often experiences severe gastrointestinal distress and diarrhea, which he attributes to "the cholera, or spasms quite as bad." He has no known surgical history. There is no documented history of chronic medical conditions.

Premorbid Personality: Mr. P was described by friends and family as a proud, vain, and imperious man who often displays a sense of entitlement that irks his relatives and friends. His family referred to letters Mr. P wrote in which he describes himself as a writer without equal and in which he frequently embroiders his accomplishments to make them sound greater than they are.

Past Psychiatric History: Mr. P described himself as "gravely traumatized" by the death of his mother and subsequent separation from his siblings. Mr. P had few friends growing up, which he attributed to his peers' jealousy of his academic and athletic prowess.

Mr. P began drinking alcohol at age 17 while at the University of Virginia. From that point on, he used alcohol regularly. His longest period of sobriety was six to eight months, during which time he was employed and happily married. His drinking often led him into rages, after which he would not remember what he had said or done. On at least one occasion, he went missing for several days and was found, amnestic and confused, wandering in the woods outside New York City. During his frequent binges, Mr. P alienated friends and family alike. Mr. P became angry when the examiner referred to his drinking, which is consistent with his family's report of his reactions to them when they voice concerns about it. Mr. P said he has tried to cut down on his alcohol intake. He also acknowledged the need for an "eye opener" most mornings.

At college, in addition to drinking, Mr. P became heavily involved in gambling, accruing a large amount of debt in just eight months' time. He asked his guardian repeatedly for money. This period marked the first strains on their relationship and set the pattern for later interactions. Mr. P had to withdraw from college due to his large debt and his guardian's refusal to pay his arrears.

During periods when Mr. P drinks heavily, he becomes depressed, finds no pleasure in his work, and is aimless. He often goes to bed for three or four days. His family noted that his dress becomes slovenly during these times, as opposed to his usual need for tidiness, and he can become malicious in his speech.

From the period of Mr. P's university years until the present admission, he has had few periods of sobriety, none lasting more than eight months at a time. His depressive episodes have followed much the same course, and although Mr. P ardently maintained that the depression comes before drinking, his family members say otherwise. In addition to lack of interest in work, poor hygiene, sleeping too much, and a deleterious change in personality, these depressive episodes of Mr. P's are marked by severe self-doubt coupled with grandiose plans to make his fortune. These plans have included publishing a world-famous periodical, speculating in real estate, and coming into an inheritance of some kind. At times, Mr. P was described as being "wild and incoherent" in his speech, more talkative than usual, and exhibiting significant psychomotor agitation. Mr. P said he never used marijuana, heroin, cocaine, or other drugs, although he once attempted suicide using laudanum. After his wife's death, Mr. P drank heavily and plunged into what he described as an "abysmal depression." His family said that during this time he often visited Virginia's burial vault late at night. He related unusual events, such as fighting a duel over a woman in France, after which a noble Scotswoman visited him daily and nursed him to health. His family denied the veracity of these events. During other episodes of heavy drinking, he would wander and be found days later, alone, confused, and feverish. Mr. P's mother-in-law would sleep near the door to intercept Mr. P if he tried to leave the house at night.

Other than having grandiose ideas, at no point did Mr. P have delusions, obsessions, compulsions, or phobias. During episodes of withdrawal from alcohol, he described frightening experiences of hearing men plot to kill him, hearing voices that plagued him no matter how far he was able to get from other people, and voices that did not answer when he spoke to them. On at least one occasion, he saw figures that others did not see, including a woman in white who addressed him in whispers. Mr. P never visited a hospital for psychiatric symptoms and has never been hospitalized for psychiatric cause. During periods of normal mood, he drinks less (if at all) and enjoys significant productivity. During these times of wellness, he excels in his professional and personal life and writes literary works to critical acclaim.

History of Present Illness: Mr. P returned to Richmond about six weeks before admission in order to raise money for his planned periodical. He resumed a romantic relationship with his first girlfriend, now widowed with two young children. He gave at least two lectures during this time on the Poetic Principle and other topics. He planned to return to New York to meet up with his mother-in-law and then return to Richmond. The night before he left Richmond, he went to a physician, sick to his stomach and feverish. The results of that visit are unknown. The next day, about one week before admission, he boarded a train for New York and stopped in Baltimore. On the day of admission, Mr. P was seen by a fellow patron in an establishment called Gunner's Tavern. Mr. P was incoherent and strangely dressed in someone else's clothes. The patron recognized the patient as Mr. Edgar Allan Poe and alerted the friend, who brought him to the hospital. He was taking no medications. The review of systems was significant for fever, chills, coughing phlegm, nausea, vomiting, headache, confusion, and dizziness.

The Discussion

Any understanding of a patient presenting with psychiatric symptoms must start with a history and mental status examination (MSE). To go beyond mere symptom identification and diagnostic classification, the evaluation must be careful, comprehensive, and systematic. The evaluation needs to include enough detail to indicate both the expression and origin of the presenting condition and any previous psychological distress. It must be obtained in a sequence that allows the clinician to consider the patient's present condition in the context of previous life experiences and personality. In clinical practice—even in the busiest of settings, such as a hospital Emergency Department (ED)—we strive to gather as much information from as many sources as possible to obtain the fullest picture of an individual's life history, beginning with the family history and moving forward in time to the history of the present illness.

There are five essential features of the systematic psychiatric evaluation: (1) a detailed history, (2) a history obtained and presented in a specific sequence, (3) a history obtained from multiple sources, (4) a systematic MSE, and (5) a careful differentiation between observations and interpretations. The remainder of this chapter will discuss each of these features in turn. By presenting Poe's "case" in two ways, we hope the reader recognizes how the first three features—regarding the history's level of detail, sequence, and source—can affect our understanding of a patient's presentation and influence our appreciation of the person experiencing the condition. Only after the clinician understands the historical aspects of an individual's suffering, can he or she proceed to examine the patient's mental state (all the while differentiating between observations and interpretations). These essential features provide the foundation from which the clinician can consider how a patient's presentation may be arising from what he has *encountered* (life story), who he *is* (dimensional), what he is *doing* (behavior), and what he *has* (disease).

A Detailed History

A detailed history, the first essential feature of the systematic psychiatric evaluation, is not unique to the *Perspectives* approach. Until recently, such a comprehensive psychiatric history, based on a format developed by Adolf Meyer (later revised by George H. Kirby and Nolan D. C. Lewis), was part of standard psychiatric teaching and practice.[1,2] This type of evaluation, requiring a focus of time and thought, is gradually being replaced—in practice if not in teaching—by one that primarily uses a checklist to screen for psychiatric conditions of a categorical nature, such as those defined by the *DSM*. This briefer evaluation typically features a history like the first one in this chapter. When applied to psychiatric conditions, this type of history reflects a general trend to reduce complex problems of thoughts, feelings, and behaviors to overly simplistic disease-like categories. Often, only those historical components most pertinent to the biological portion of the biopsychosocial model[3] are used to assess psychiatric conditions, and this is commonly done by the patients themselves via a variety of self-rating forms for psychiatric conditions. This trend toward a less comprehensive history may be related to the benefit of brevity (appealing to clinicians working under the constraints of managed health care) and to the wide availability of pharmacologic treatments for categorically diagnosed psychiatric conditions (appealing to clinicians and patients in the setting of the cultural influence of the pharmaceutical industry and the *DSM*).

A Sequential History

To think about psychiatric conditions in a way that pushes past these cultural pressures and permits complete formulations and thoughtful recommendations, the clinician needs a comprehensive history. And, although a comprehensive history is necessary for the systematic psychiatric evaluation, it is not sufficient. The sequence of the history itself, beginning with the family history and moving forward in time, is the second integral component of the systematic psychiatric evaluation. This sequential unfolding of the patient's life allows appreciation of the patient as an individual (and how different individuals in different circumstances respond to life's challenges) and enriches understanding of the patient's condition. The sequence of the history presented in version two makes it much less likely that the clinician will understand the patient's present condition as emerging simply from the pressure of his present circumstances. Using the chronological history presented in version two, the clinician's diagnostic thinking is biased less toward excessive focus on the chief complaint and present illness as the primary explanation for the patient's current symptoms. For example, similarly to Poe, a patient may present malodorous and disheveled, with the chief complaint of intoxication and a history of alcohol use and low mood. A clinician—whether a psychiatrist or primary care physician—can become habituated to the superficial similarity of such presentations and begin to think that all patients with this presentation are the same, which of course they are not. As in the case of Poe, the lack of recognition of the patient's individuality can lead the clinician to neglect critical aspects of the personal and psychiatric history. When first getting to know patients, it is best to keep one's thinking broad and open. Thus, taking a comprehensive history and recording it in the medical record in a specific sequence are essential features of the psychiatric evaluation. A more complete formulation of the case and treatment plan for the patient naturally arises from such a detailed narrative (refer to appendix A for a sample history format).

Multiple Sources of Information

The third essential feature of the systematic psychiatric evaluation is historical information obtained from multiple sources—individuals (e.g., family members, friends, physicians) who know the patient or some aspect of the patient's condition well. The primary purpose is to expand on and enhance the history provided by the patient, whose point of view may be limited and/or skewed due to a variety of psychiatric conditions. In the case of Poe, for example, childhood conflicts, demoralization, alcohol dependence, depressed mood, and intoxication could all potentially affect his recounting of his life story and make aspects of the history—whether provided by the patient or by other informants—inaccurate. For example, Poe's intoxication could lead him to distort memories of past feelings (such as being "gravely traumatized" over the death of his mother) or events (such as the duel over the woman in France). Or, frustration with Poe's difficult moods and behaviors could prompt a cousin to accuse Poe of frequently embroidering his accomplishments to make them sound greater than they are.

Information obtained from a variety of sources helps the clinician understand how others see the patient and his history, and allows the clinician to form a more complete understanding of the patient's condition. From our experience evaluating patients previously assessed by other clinicians, we have found that gathering information from additional sources is not routinely practiced. Yet, it needs to be an essential feature of the systematic psychiatric evaluation of every patient in every practice setting. The clinician is encouraged to find an appropriate way of including an outside informant in every evaluation, including the instance of an adult seeking individual outpatient psychotherapy. In fact, individual psychotherapy provided to a person whose history is not well understood is hampered from the outset and represents a risk to the patient and family. In our experience, most patients and their family members are receptive to and appreciative of these discussions. In the course of our careers we have not always made these contacts as part of the initial evaluation, but—over time—have come to appreciate their value in understanding a patient's troubles.

Approach Influences Formulation

We presented two versions of the Poe case to highlight the first three essential features of the systematic psychiatric evaluation: a detailed history obtained and presented in a specific sequence, with historical information gathered from multiple sources. We do not know all the details of Edgar Allan Poe's medical history, life story, or cause of death. It is not our intent to use this case to provide a psychiatric formulation of this illustrious literary figure. We present two versions of Poe's case to demonstrate how the way we approach a psychiatric evaluation can influence our formulation of the case. In the first version, which focuses primarily on the chief complaint and history of present illness, Poe can be readily diagnosed with an alcohol use disorder and perhaps a depressive disorder, but our understanding of the temporal and causal relationship between these psychiatric conditions is limited. Only in the second history, where we learn from Poe's family that his depression actually came after drinking (contrary to what he maintained), did we obtain information that could be used to support the formulation that Poe's alcohol use is the primary problem and the disorder from which any depressive symptoms are secondarily arising. And, although both versions contain enough family history to suggest the possible influence of genetics on the initiation and maintenance of Poe's alcohol use, the second version, with its level of detail, sequence, and use of collateral information, enables us to consider the additional role that early life losses, such as his mother's death and his separation from siblings, as well as later academic and financial struggles may play in sustaining his drinking. Similarly, the second version's use of information gathered from outside sources allows us to better understand aspects of Poe's enduring personality, such as his high intelligence and apparent sense of self-importance and entitlement. With this fuller understanding, we are in a better position to consider the role of his intelligence and temperament in the psychiatric formulation. Although this might not be of greatest relevance to assessing and treating the condition with which he presented to the ED, an understanding of the dimensions of his personality would be essential to any longitudinal treatment.

A Systematic Mental Status Examination

The fourth essential feature of the psychiatric evaluation is a systematic MSE. We did not examine Poe, of course, and there is no record of a complete examination of his mental state at the time of his ED presentation, so we are unable to present this component of the evaluation here. However, we would like to discuss briefly some of the components of a systematic MSE, emphasizing first that the MSE is not simply a recitation

TABLE 2.1   *Components of the Mental Status Examination (MSE)*

1. Appearance/Behavior	5. Content of Thought
2. Speech	Delusions
Volume	Obsessions
Rate	Compulsions
Rhythm	Phobias
Fluidity	6. Insight and Judgment
Spontaneity	7. Cognition
Latency	Level of consciousness
Thought disorder	Orientation
3. Mood and Affect (observed and reported)	Memory
Stability, reactivity, appropriateness	Praxis
Vital sense	Language
Self-attitude	Abstraction
Thoughts of death, suicide, homicide	Fund of knowledge
4. Abnormal Perceptions	Attention
Illusions	Calculation
Hallucinations	Executive function

Source: Adapted with permission from Lyketsos CG, *Psychiatric Aspects of Neurologic Diseases—Practical Approaches to Patient Care*. Oxford, 2008.

of different *DSM* criteria. (As mentioned, a more complete discussion of the MSE, including a version to be used at the "bedside," can be found in appendix B.) Rather, it is a systematic and structured assessment of the patient's current thoughts, feelings, and behaviors using a question-and-answer format. The MSE reveals information about the patient's mental life just as the physical examination reveals information about the patient's organ systems. It is not, however, an exercise in free association. Although we do not wish to lead the patient to provide specific answers to our questions, we must make it clear what we need to understand. Only the patient's conscious feelings and thoughts are being examined (no one, not even a psychiatrist, can examine the patient's unconscious mental processes). One purpose of this empathic conversation with the patient is to help the clinician understand what it is like to be walking in the patient's shoes, while at the same time deciding whether his mental experiences meet *a priori* definitions of psychopathologic phenomena (e.g., hallucinations, delusions, obsessions), such as the ones found in *Sims' Symptoms in the Mind*.[4] In addition to assessing the patient's conscious experiences, the MSE assesses certain cognitive capacities.

A comprehensive MSE might take 20 to 30 minutes. This is not dissimilar to the amount of time that would be spent conducting any careful physical or neurologic examination. The examination should be conducted in a systematic way to avoid missing any accessible psychiatric phenomena—just as cardiac auscultation is performed in a certain sequence to examine all accessible areas of the heart. Beginning psychiatrists are at times concerned about the reliability of the MSE. We would like to reassure them that, when this examination is conducted carefully by a skilled clinician, it is as reliable as any physical examination, including cardiac auscultation.

Observations before Interpretations

The fifth and final essential feature of the systematic psychiatric evaluation is careful differentiation between observations and interpretations. This is a more subtle feature and one that can be challenging for beginning clinicians to grasp. However, its application is critical to a successful evaluation. In compiling Poe's case, we sought to distinguish the observable phenomena that lay entangled with interpretations written by literary scholars and historians[5] and to include only observations—either of internal phenomena as reported by Poe himself or of external phenomena observed by others—in the case presentations. As we have previously articulated[6] and will illustrate in case 4 in part 2, patients and clinicians have a natural tendency to use meaningful connections to explain mental life and behavior. Explaining our thoughts, feelings, and behaviors by telling a story and using meaningful connections (interpretations) is a distinctly human way of making sense of our experiences. However, these interpretations are not always correct and can lead us down false pathways, which may not always be helpful or adaptive. When a clinician asks a patient about an event, thoughts, feelings, or behaviors, the patient may respond with a mixture of observations and interpretations. For example:

Clinician: "How is your energy?"
Patient: "I have been drinking a lot more coffee during the day and so have had trouble sleeping at night, and then I feel tired the next day."

Contrast the previous patient response with the following one, in which the patient resists giving meaning to observations about her behavior:

Patient: "I have been feeling tired for a while, I've also been drinking more coffee during the day and waking up a lot more frequently at night."

In taking the history and performing the MSE, a clinician must be vigilant to distinguish between observations and interpretations. And, again, separating these from each other is not an easy matter. As stated previously, humans tend to connect phenomena in our daily lives in a way that gives meaning to experience. This is an overlearned skill that a clinician must unlearn to be effective in the evaluation and treatment of patients who present with psychiatric symptoms. Once the clinician has clarified the patient's observations regarding past and current phenomena (events, thoughts, feelings, and behaviors) with the help of outside informants (for events and behaviors) to ensure an accurate history and valid MSE, then he or she can begin the formulation. Regardless of the formulation, the patient's explanations for past and current events, thoughts, feelings, and behaviors must not be discounted; at times, however, they may need to be placed in the proper context. For example, a person saying that his poor work performance caused his low mood may, instead, be performing poorly at work due to his low mood. The patient would need education regarding the effect of depressive disorder on energy and concentration to help him better understand the *setting* and *sequence* (and the causal chain) of the illness.

Summary

Although it is tempting to put forth our formulation of the case of Poe, we will not do so here. The purpose of part 1 of this book is to illustrate key concepts. In this chapter we have used the Poe case to demonstrate the rationale for the *Perspectives* approach to the history. Each subsequent chapter in part 1 will use a case to illuminate the key concepts underlying each of the four perspectives. Thus, part 1 of the book, including this chapter, does not provide formulations for the cases. However, each case in part 2 will contain a full formulation to demonstrate what a *Perspectives*-informed formulation is and what it is not (it is not, for example, simply writing down the *DSM* multiaxial diagnoses or listing biopsychosocial factors).

We hope we have demonstrated how important a detailed, sequenced, well-informed, and observation-based history and MSE are in working with patients who have psychiatric conditions. The history and MSE are the basis for everything that follows and are essential in applying the *Perspectives* approach to psychiatric conditions.

Summary Points
Essential features of the systematic psychiatric evaluation:

1 A detailed history

2 A history obtained and presented in a specific sequence

3 A history obtained from multiple sources

4 A systematic MSE

5 A careful differentiation between observations and interpretations

CHAPTER THREE

The Life-Story Perspective

It has been said that grief is a kind of madness. I disagree. There is a sanity to grief, in its just proportion of emotion to cause, that madness does not have.

—from *Nothing Was the Same*, by Kay Redfield Jamison

In this chapter and all subsequent chapters, we begin by presenting the case, in dialogue format, followed by a structured discussion of the topic at hand (in this case, the life-story perspective), and concluding with a few key summary points.

The Case

D r. Gabriel meets Ms. T, a 59-year-old woman, who presents to his outpatient practice for help in coping with her husband's recent death.

(Dr. Gabriel's comments are printed in *italics*.)

Hi, Ms. T. I'm sorry to be meeting you under these circumstances. How are you doing?

Not good, I think. Everybody is telling me things will get better, but nothing has—and it's been two months now. We'd been together 40 years . . . and then he got leukemia. (Ms. T's eyes well up with tears.)

I'm so sorry.

It's still unbelievable to me that he's gone. Nick had only been really sick for the last year. I think I'm still in shock. I've never known anyone who's died, except my grandparents. Even my parents are still alive.

Why don't you start by telling me more about your parents.

They're in Rockport, Maine. That's where I grew up. They both turn 80 this year. Mom's terrific. She stayed at home with all of us and now just dotes on Dad. He's still working part time, believe it or not—still goes into his law office every day.

Do you have any brothers or sisters?

I've got an older sister, Amy, we're just sixteen months apart. She divorced years ago and never did remarry.

Anyone else besides you and Amy?

There's three of us altogether. Jim's the baby, he's 51. He's divorced, but he got married again right away.

(Ms. T is asked about her extended and immediate family's physical and mental health and she reports that, besides hypertension in her father, there have been no problems. Ms. T is also asked about and denies any problems during her own gestation, infancy, and childhood.)

What year did you graduate from high school?

1959. But I stayed at home and went to junior college before transferring to St. John's College. I loved Annapolis so much I never left.

Did you date in college?

That's when I met my husband; he was a midshipman. We got married in the Academy Chapel my senior year and I got pregnant right away. I stayed at home with both my boys—they're two years apart—until the younger one started high school. That's when I went back to school for nursing, and I've been working med-surg in the same hospital ever since. I love my job.

Are your sons nearby?

Chris, he's in Pennsylvania, but the younger one—Arnie—he's got a place here in Annapolis.

Any grandchildren?

Not yet, although Chris is finally engaged. He's a pediatrician, so I know he's been busy. Arnie's gay and not seeing anyone now. He's been a big help to me.

Do you drink or smoke?

I might have a glass of white wine if I'm out to dinner. I don't drink anything at home. I've never smoked.

And have you used any drugs?

No, never.

And you live here in Annapolis?

We've got a house right on the water, about a mile from the hospital. Before Nick got sick, we were planning to retire, maybe in California—that's where he's from—after the house was paid off. There's only five more years left on the mortgage. (Ms. T starts to well up again.)

What did your husband do after leaving the Naval Academy?

He never left the Navy! He was an engineer for them.

(Ms. T is asked about and denies any medical conditions, surgeries, medications, and drug allergies.)

I'd like to switch gears now and ask some questions about what you're usually like as a person. For instance, I'm wondering if you're the kind of person who usually sees the glass as half empty or half full.

Oh, I'm a total optimist, or was until recently.

What kinds of things do you usually enjoy doing?

Well, Nick and I used to bowl in a league. That was a lot of fun. And I've always tried to keep a neat, well, let's say "perfect" house. I think I get that from my mother. And I used to help Nick out with the yard. That garden was his pride and joy. (Ms. T begins welling up.)

Have you been spending any time with friends?

A little, now that the weather is getting nicer. They tried to get me to go to a support group for widows and widowers, but everyone seemed so much older . . . it made me feel even more depressed.

Do you usually like being around people?

Oh, yes. I love being around people, especially the young people at work. I still feel like I'm a positive person. It's just hard right now.

*You said you were Catholic, right?**

I was raised Catholic, but Nick's Lutheran, and we went to a Lutheran church. But, since he died, I've been going to Catholic mass and I think I'm going to go back to the church. It's comforting to me. (With the patient's permission, Dr. Gabriel talked, via telephone, to Ms.

*As noted in the preface, these cases are presented in an abridged, dialogue format. Thus, no single case represents a complete rendering of any particular patient's history as originally obtained.

T's younger son, who confirms Ms. T's description of herself. He says his mother is usually quite cheerful and positive, has a stable group of friends, and enjoys a number of social activities. He agrees that his mother has been sad since his father died, but says that he's been encouraged that she's felt up to seeing friends and has been able to take care of herself and the house, in addition to going back to work. He adds, "Mom's never been on her own as an adult, and I think she just misses Dad's company and is finding it hard to do things alone.")

Ms. T, you mentioned that you've never seen a psychiatrist before; have you ever wanted to or thought you needed to?

No, I've really had a good life.

So, let's go back now to talk about your husband's illness. When was he first diagnosed?

Well, that was about a year ago, but—looking back—he'd been feeling tired for at least three months before that. He said it was just "old age," but I finally got him to come see one of our docs. They did a blood test and knew pretty much right away it was leukemia. And from there, Nick was in and out of the hospital with chemo and infections and all the rest. Three months after his diagnosis, his oncologist told me he probably wouldn't live more than a year. And he was right. He made it about nine more months. He was in home hospice for the last three months. That was the toughest time. There was a nurse's aide during the day, but I was only getting about four or five hours of sleep. There was so much to take care of: dealing with the legal stuff, bathing him, trying to get him to eat. And I was still working—eventually I took a leave of absence, the last month or so. It was just exhausting physically and mentally, watching him just slowly deteriorate like that. (Ms. T's eyes fill with tears.)

You miss him . . .

Yes. I feel so alone without him. He was my best friend.

I'm glad you're here. How are you sleeping now?

I sometimes wake up at night, thinking about how much I miss him. I've even dreamed about him.

And your appetite for food, how has that been?

I couldn't eat much right after he died, but that's getting better. It's hard to cook for just one person.

And your sex drive: any thoughts or interest?

None.

Have you noticed any changes in your energy level or concentration?

A little bit. I feel I'm getting back to normal at work now, but when I come home at night I'm really pooped. I'm so busy at work that I really don't have any time to think about anything else.

MSE: Ms. T is a well-groomed, alert, and cooperative woman who appears her stated age. She is easily engaged in conversation, making good eye contact. She is tearful at times when talking about her late husband. Ms. T sits quietly and demonstrates no tics or tremor. She responds to questions without delay. Speech is normal in rate, amount, and volume. It is not circumstantial and there is no evidence of thought disorder or aphasia. Ms. T describes her mood as "Sad. I miss him terribly." She appears euthymic during some of the interview, but looks sad when talking about her husband and her feelings of loss. Ms. T denies feeling guilty. She is optimistic about the future and feels good about herself. She denies any suicidal or homicidal thoughts, but says she sometimes wonders what death is like or how her death would be handled by loved ones. Ms. T denies any hallucinations, delusions, obsessions, compulsions, or phobias. She is fully oriented and has a good fund of information, with a Mini-Mental State Exam (MMSE)[1] score of 30/30. Her intelligence is above average and her insight and judgment are normal.

The Discussion

In chapter 1, we introduced the four perspectives in a particular order, beginning with the disease perspective. We did this because the disease perspective is most familiar to students of medicine, as most nonpsychiatric medical conditions are best understood as diseases (that is, a clinical syndrome arising from a broken part via a pathophysiologic process). However, in this chapter and the rest of the book we will begin with the life-story perspective, as this is the sequence in which the four perspectives are best applied to patients (and as they will be applied in part 2).

Why start with the life-story perspective when evaluating patients? Because the life story is the most natural, and personal, way of explaining someone's thoughts, feelings, and behaviors. We grow up hearing and telling stories; we were story tellers long before we became patients and/

or clinicians. A story is not merely a chronological listing of events but a narrative in which particular events occurring in the life of an individual are understood to account for that individual's state of mind and behavior. The elements of a life story—a *sequence* of events occurring in the *setting* of a person's life that produces psychological and behavioral *outcomes*—are the same whether the story is about a fictional character (e.g., Hamlet), a historical figure (e.g., Poe), or a patient (e.g., Ms. T).

Setting ——————→ Sequence ——————→ Outcome...

We also start with the life-story perspective because it is in the *context* of an individual's life story that personality dimensions arise and any behavioral disorders and/or psychiatric diseases occur. (Although these other dimensions and conditions occur in the context of a life story, this does not mean that the life story is the cause of these other psychiatric conditions, or vice versa, for that matter.)

The life story consists of the psychological products of an individual's personal *encounters*. It is the perspective that is unique to the individual so, in thinking about the psychiatric condition of each patient, we begin with this perspective. Examples of the kinds of psychological outcome that follow a personal *encounter* and prompt an individual to seek psychiatric attention are grief, frustration, disconnection, anger, guilt, and shame. The life-story perspective encourages us to think about a patient's psychiatric condition as originating from something she has *encountered* (versus the disease perspective, in which a problem arises from something an individual *has*). In Ms. T's case, her flourishing life is painfully sidetracked by the loss of her husband. Ms. T's grieving disrupts her life course, and she seeks psychiatric help to grapple with the unfamiliar feelings and thoughts she is experiencing after her husband's death.

As described in chapter 1, the life-story perspective, with its logic of narrative—*setting, sequence*, and *outcome*—encourages a clinician to use the story method to help a patient respond to an event. Different versions of life stories—Freudian, Jungian, etc.—can be told, but the type of story told is less important than the therapeutic relationship and other factors.[2] As we saw in chapter 2, by taking a detailed history in the recommended *sequence*, a clinician is able to understand empathically both the *setting* in which the event/response occurs and the personality of the patient to whom the event is occurring and from whom the response is emanating. For example, when a natural disaster strikes a community, individual responses can range from resignation to devastation, according to the individual's past experiences and personality. (The complex interactions between the perspectives and how they affect formulation and treatment will be discussed in more detail in part 2.) In Ms. T's case, life was going well before her husband's diagnosis and subsequent death. She is a generally stable woman for whom the expected psychological outcome after her husband's death is grief. Grief responses are primarily emotional but also can color an individual's thoughts and alter her behavior. Certain kinds of thoughts (e.g., preoccupation with the deceased) and behaviors (e.g., disturbed sleeping and eating) are as much a part of the reaction as are certain kinds of moods.

Grieving is an immediate and understandable psychological reaction to the death of someone close to a person. Although Ms. T's grief is what prompts her to seek psychiatric treatment, not everyone who experiences the death of a loved one becomes a patient. Indeed, most people adapt without psychiatric help to even the most significant events, including such a loss as Ms. T experienced. The patient who does present to a clinician for help is usually feeling overwhelmed by the event that has intruded into her life. Such an event can disrupt, or threaten to disrupt, concrete plans—such as retirement and relocation—but it can also cause a patient to question her hopes and dreams, as Ms. T describes happening to her. This state of being overwhelmed with loneliness, as Ms. T experiences after the death of her husband of forty years, is best characterized as demoralization.[2] Its treatment is the creation of a story, by clinician and patient together, from the psychotherapeutic relationship—the goal of which is to restore the patient to a state of mastery. *Rescripting* a patient's narrative in this way is the goal of treatment for any psychiatric condition that has arisen from what a patient has encountered.

Stories are central to the way humans communicate. They explain things that causal mechanisms cannot. For instance, we may grasp through cognitive neuroscience the associations of brain states with emotion and eventually come to identify the parts of the brain essential to the experience of grief. We might even statistically predict what losses evoke and sustain grief sensations. But only the *personal* story will allow us to make sense of and explain the meaning of an individual's grieving. While neuroscience may someday reveal how emotional responses arise, it will remain unable to provide a framework that grasps why *for a specific individual in a particular situation* certain emotional expressions are appropriate while others are not. Anthropology and sociology are better able to provide such insight[3] in a way that neuroscience cannot. Stories and the understanding they transmit differ inherently from the "broken parts" of most diseases. Stories, in contrast to the causal explanations of diseases, transmit an understanding that does not so much discover a truth as propose one. This truth is offered in the therapy to be either recognized by the patient as "fitting" the significance and implications of her emotions (now framed as apt outcomes to the *setting* and *sequence* in which she has lived) or rejected to await a new proposed truth. This creation of a story together conveys to the patient that, although you can't feel her loss in the same way that you feel your own (or that she feels hers), you can feel something like what she feels.

The extent of Ms. T's grief at the loss of her husband is a normal emotional reaction after the death of a close loved one, which sometimes prompts an individual, as it did in Ms. T's case, to seek psychiatric help. We present Ms. T's story to illustrate the key components of the life-story perspective. Her grief following the death of her husband represents a disturbance in feelings and thoughts to which life-story reasoning can be readily applied. It is a psychological experience with which many readers may be familiar and to which they can relate.

In the *setting* of a loss like the one that struck Ms. T, most people have a predictable *sequence* of psychological *outcomes*: emotional numbness (or, as Ms. T said, "shock"), followed by disbelief (it has been two months since her husband died, but she says she still can't believe he is gone), and recurrent memories of the deceased (in Ms. T's case, these thoughts usually come at night). These memories evoke feelings of sorrow, longing, love, and loss and are often accompanied by "wellings" of sadness and crying. The memories and feelings intrude intermittently and unpredictably into one's day and then recede. For Ms. T, these episodes are less likely to occur when she is busy at work and are evident during the evaluation. The unique mixture of feelings, their bittersweet nature, and their brief duration in the wake of such a loss all help to distinguish the sadness of grief from depression. Other phenomena, such as disrupted sleep, appetite, and daily activity, might be found in both major depressive disorder and grief. In Ms. T's case, she describes mild problems with sleep and appetite, especially initially, and she also notes a change in her sex drive. Ms. T is taking comfort in her childhood faith and, although lonely, is generally hopeful. But because Ms. T is still feeling overwhelmed by her grieving two months after her husband's death (a lack of resiliency that was uncharacteristic for her), she seeks psychiatric treatment.

We hope that, with the help of Ms. T's personal story, we have demonstrated the underlying conceptual triad of the life-story perspective. The key elements of the life-story perspective, like any narrative, are *setting, sequence,* and *outcome.* The clinician must understand what a patient has *encountered* and how it has affected her (in part by understanding who she is as a person). Once this understanding is achieved, the clinician can help the patient *rescript* a personal narrative that is more effective, active, and optimistic.

Summary Points

The life-story perspective:

1 Is a personal perspective

2 Is based on the logic of narrative with its triad of *setting, sequence,* and *outcome,* which is produced meaningfully and understandably

3 It applies to psychiatric conditions that arise from something an individual has *encountered*

4 It suggests *rescripting* as the treatment goal

CHAPTER FOUR

The Dimensional Perspective

Variability is the law of life, and as no two faces are the same, so
no two bodies are alike, and no two individuals react alike and
behave alike under the abnormal conditions which we know as
disease.

—from William Osler's *On the Educational Value of the Medical Society*

The Case

Dr. Sen meets RJ, a 19-year-old male, accompanied by his mother
for an initial evaluation in a community psychiatry program for
patients who have special needs. RJ's mother, Ms. J, brings him for evaluation due to a recurrence in behavior problems at school. Because RJ has
limited verbal ability, the history is obtained from his mother.

(Dr. Sen's comments are printed in *italics*.)

Hi, RJ. I'm going to talk some with your mother first, okay?
(RJ nods his assent.)

*Ms. J, thanks for getting RJ's records sent to us. I've reviewed them
but will go over them again with you today to make sure they're all
correct from your point of view. I know from the records that RJ has
been seen by a psychiatrist before, for similar problems.*

Yes, that was back in Raleigh. He's always been good at home, but
at school he can have some kind of temper tantrum! Yes, indeed.

*I understand from his previous evaluations that he's got an older
sister.*

Yes, but she doesn't have any of RJ's problems. She's here in Memphis. That's why me and RJ moved. She's married now and has a baby on the way.

And the records say she was never depressed, but that other people in your family have been treated for depression. Is that right?

Well, that's not on my side of the family, but RJ's daddy's. RJ's daddy's brother was depressed. Both of them seemed depressed to me. RJ's daddy died when RJ was a little baby. He had sugar.

What kind of work did he do?

He was a handyman, and a hard worker. He made a good life for us, considering.

Considering?

That he didn't go that far in school—he only went to the sixth grade. He had to quit school to work. He was good at fixing things, though, and could even do electric.

What about you? How far were you able to go in school?

I graduated. I got a good job working at a school as a nurse's aide.

That must have been hard—working and raising RJ and his sister by yourself.

It was hard at times, but I've been truly blessed. I come from a big family and my brothers and sisters have always been there for me. And my church—I'm Baptist.

You're from North Carolina, right? Is that where RJ was born?

Yes.

Anything remarkable about your pregnancy with him or his birth?

Not a bit. Everything was normal as can be. He was 8 pounds, 2 ounces, and healthy as a horse. Everything was fine until it came time for him to start talking.

Tell me about that.

Well, that's when I knew that something must be wrong. His sister started talking a blue streak when she was just 1 year old. But RJ was going on 3 and hadn't said more than a word or two. We took him for his 3-year-old checkup—he was never sick, so we just took him in for his shots—and his doctor knew then that something was wrong. We got him into speech therapy, and he talks now but he'll never be normal, we know.

That must be sad for you.

Of course it is, but it could be worse. RJ's a handful at times, but we all love him. Even his teachers say he's got the biggest heart! He's at the same school since he was 4; that is, until this year, when we moved here. He's taking the bus now every day, and I'm always here when he gets home. Bless him, he can't use a key to let himself in.

I saw that RJ last had IQ testing about two years ago.

I asked for him to be tested again. The others had been done in school. This one wasn't any different from the others, though.

It said his IQ was 49.

Right. "Moderate," they say. See, it could be worse. He's able to do a lot of things himself. He gets dressed, except for tying his shoes, by himself. He likes to watch TV and can even read some of the *TV Guide*. He knows how to write his name. RJ's main problem is he doesn't like to be told what to do—especially now. I mean he's a grown man. When they tell him to do something at this school and he doesn't want to do it, he throws a fit.

A temper tantrum?

Yes indeed. I let him do most whatever he wants at home—which is mainly watching TV—and he usually doesn't give me any problems. He might stomp his feet or whine when I ask him to do one of his chores, like sweeping the floor, but he minds me. But at school, it's a different story. I guess they put a lot more things on him, and he doesn't know a soul there. If they tell him to do something, like stop pestering someone, then he gets all mad and throws himself on the floor and starts kicking and he gets himself all worked up. Or if he's having a hard time reading or doing a problem in his school book, that will set him off. They even had to take him to the emergency room once because he was in such a state. That happened a couple of times back in Raleigh, too, but years ago.

But he's never been hospitalized?

No, they just gave him a shot to calm him down, and then I took him home and he was fine. He saw a psychiatrist back in Raleigh, but they didn't start him on any regular medication. They just said keep doing what we were doing. Like I say, he's pretty good at home and was doing better at school, and then I moved us here to be closer to my new grandbaby when she comes. And RJ's having some trouble adjusting to the change.

MSE: RJ is a well-groomed, neatly dressed, alert, and cooperative young man who is slender and appears slightly younger than his stated age. He has no dysplastic features. He is able to run and jump in place. He demonstrates no tics or tremor, but is a bit fidgety. RJ is cooperative, but speaks softly and his speech is dysarthric. RJ occasionally repeats what his mother says. He also talks to himself and laughs. RJ is able to respond to some direct questions in a goal-oriented fashion, but only in two- to three-word utterances. At times, RJ uses hand gestures to communicate. He knows his new address but not his telephone number. RJ is unable to describe his mood without prompts, but when asked if he is "happy" or "sad," he endorses happy, and he appears to be cheerful. There is no evidence of self-injurious behavior, hallucinations, delusions, compulsions, or phobias. He knows the day of the week, month, and year. His MMSE score is 12/30, with 6 points deducted for orientation, 5 for attention/calculation, 2 for recall, and 5 for language/praxis.

The Discussion

In this chapter, we present a case of intellectual disability (ID) to demonstrate the central conceptual triad of the dimensional perspective. Just as human beings vary dimensionally in physical attributes, such as height and weight, they also vary dimensionally in psychological characteristics. In the dimensional perspective, the underlying conceptual triad is that an aspect of a person's psychological dimensions represents a *potential* vulnerability for certain life events to *provoke* in that person an emotional *response*.

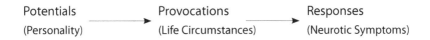

Potentials	Provocations	Responses
(Personality)	(Life Circumstances)	(Neurotic Symptoms)

The dimensional perspective encourages us to think about a patient's psychiatric condition, like RJ's, as originating in psychological dimensions, or who the patient *is*.

Psychological dimensions (like intelligence or independence) are present and measureable in every individual. These dimensions are graded such that a particular individual can have the same, more of, or less of the feature when compared to others. In populations the dimension can be represented on axes (as in the IQ curve), with any specific individual occupying a specific, and relatively stable, point on the dimension. Thinking about psychological dimensions as occurring along a continuum, as dimensions, helps us understand an individual's *potential* strengths and vulnerabilities in particular circumstances. For instance, someone who is intelligent and emotionally dependent may breeze through an organic chemistry course but become overwhelmed by a romantic break-up. Another student who is less bright but more happy-go-lucky may struggle to pass organic chemistry but will deal with a romantic loss without difficulty.

A problematic response develops only when a potentially vulnerable individual (vulnerable because of where he is on a given dimension) meets a particular stress or provocation (one with the capacity to expose the vulnerability),[1] which may or may not spur the individual to seek professional help. An awareness of the patient's position along psychological dimensions helps us understand the origin of the problematic thoughts, feelings, and behavioral choices and informs treatment for those, like RJ, who do seek help.

The reader may be less familiar with this dimensional approach to personality, with its roots in psychology, because most clinicians, including psychologists, do not currently use it. The standard clinical approach used in the *DSM* is typological rather than dimensional. Although the *DSM*'s typological approach has reliability (between personality disorder "clusters") and some research utility, we have found it to be less helpful for clinical care.

Many patients come to treatment because they are having difficulty navigating the ups and downs of everyday life related to dimensional vulnerabilities. Some are experiencing trouble for the first time in the face of a novel life event. In RJ's case, he had been doing relatively well managing his life's demands, despite moderately severe ID, until he changed schools. As RJ adjusts to the new school environment, we anticipate his behavioral difficulties will recede. Happily, RJ is not one of the few patients who come for treatment because of a severe psychological vulnerability and a longstanding pattern of difficulties with familiar life events. Nevertheless, regardless of a patient's position along a dimension, these psychological dimensions inform who a person is: the *potential* to emotionally *respond* either positively or negatively to a particular *provocation*, including medical or psychiatric disease.

In this chapter, we present a case of subnormal intelligence to introduce the psychological dimensions. We have found that learners are better able to grasp the key concepts of the dimensional perspective when they are first presented in the context of intelligence. Modeling the most obvious example of problematic cognitive dimensions—low intelligence—clarifies the more-difficult-to-grasp dimensions of temperament. Once modeled in this way and applied to the case presented here, these same points will be illustrated (in part 2) in cases of vulnerable temperaments.

As described in chapter 1, the key concepts of the dimensional perspective are *potential* (where a particular individual stands on the relevant dimension), *provocation* (the specific circumstance of a poor fit for the individual), and *response* (the specific behaviors or feelings that result from the poor fit). In the dimensional perspective, the driving force for a patient's psychiatric condition is the poor fit between who the person is and the circumstances in which that person finds himself. Two distinct general psychological dimensions can be measured in individuals and populations: cognition and temperament. For both dimensions, the emotional responses that have the potential to be provoked in response to life events are similar and include sadness, aggression, discouragement, and anxiety. In the present case, RJ's stomping his feet, whining, kicking, and throwing himself on the floor when he is unable to perform certain tasks or when he is asked to redirect his attention or activities most likely are behavioral expressions of frustration, discouragement, and anger.

The overarching goal of treatment for all types of responses related to dimensional vulnerabilities is guidance, and the overarching goal assumes that the specific treatment goals differ only in what the clinician is guiding the patient toward. For individuals who have subnormal intelligence, the therapeutic focus may be education and employment. In some cases, the specific treatment goal may be to guide the patient to a different educational setting; in others, to lower educational and career goals, and so on. RJ, at home and in his special education environment, has been guided gently to learn and master various life skills, such as how to dress and groom independently, to read well enough to choose TV programs, and to write his name. Both his home and school settings are highly supportive, nurturing environments where care has been taken to gradually teach RJ these skills to avoid overwhelming his intelligence and causing frustration.

Despite these efforts, it is impossible to always present the ideal, perfectly pitched challenge to RJ. At home and at school, demands have been placed on him that are, at times, followed by behavior outbursts. One of RJ's home chores is sweeping the floor. Sometimes he can do this without protest and sometimes he can't. Part of the clinician's job is to sort out whether RJ's behavior is coming from an overly challenging demand or from what RJ's temperament is bringing to the demand at a certain time. Once that is understood, the treatment can focus on either adjusting the demand or guiding the patient with alternative ways of coping with emotions in the face of the demand. Although RJ has not yet finished school, the skills that he has been able to learn through such home and educational guidance are helping to prepare him for more independent living and for sheltered employment. For temperament vulnerabilities, the aim is to anticipate, manage, develop better ways of coping with, and, if necessary and possible, avoid potential provocations.

We have chosen to use the cognitive psychological dimension of intelligence as the model for understanding the dimensional perspective because it is the most obvious. It is the aspect of human mental life that has been the best-studied and understood in relationship both to its measurement and to the troubles that the problematic dispositions, particularly low IQ, bring. Thus, the history and implications of this cognitive dimension have been widely disseminated and now seem self-evident to us. Intelligence is a universal, measurable psychological feature that can be represented in a graded fashion within a population. The psychological dimensions (cognition and temperament) have multiple determinants, however, and so can be affected by disease or behaviors, which may themselves have genetic and environmental determinants. IQ, for example, is not distributed evenly on a bell-shaped curve. Rather there is an increase on the left side of the curve representing individuals who have brain-injuring conditions, some of which may be reversible and others of which are permanent. For instance, in this case, the patient has some symptoms of a pervasive developmental disorder, like autism, which can be associated with intellectual disability. Other examples of disease affecting a psychological dimension are Down syndrome and Alzheimer disease (which may reduce intelligence) and major depression (which may decrease or increase emotional reactivity).

Individuals who have ID have a higher incidence of emotional and

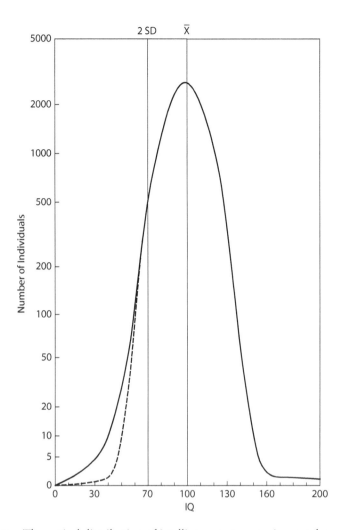

FIGURE 4.1. Theoretical distribution of intelligence test scores in a total population (X = mean, SD = standard deviation). *Source:* Adapted from Penrose LS. *The Biology of Mental Defect*, 3rd ed. London: Sidgwick and Jackson, 1963.

behavioral problems (50%) than peers without ID (18%),[2] a phenomenon seen in RJ, who initially came to psychiatric attention due to behavioral problems at school. The emotional responses of cognitively challenged individuals do not differ qualitatively from those of individuals without ID. Like all individuals who have vulnerabilities to certain provocations, the usual repertoire of emotional responses includes aggression, anxiety, sadness, demoralization, frustration, and other unpleasant states. In this case, due to RJ's limited verbal ability, we can infer from the *setting* and *sequence* in which they have occurred only that they represent a behavioral expression of emotions. RJ could possibly be feeling angry at being redirected in his activities, anxious about being in a new home and school environment, sad about being separated from his previous classmates and teachers, and frustrated with his inability to perform certain cognitive and/or motor tasks. Many of these responses in individuals who have ID or other vulnerabilities disappear from clinical sight as the individuals mature and are able to adapt more successfully to life's demands and circumstances. In RJ's case, they had been improving over the past two years. However, problems may re-arise with new provocations, as they did for RJ, such as relocation with its changes in social contacts and routines. In this case, as is typical, the individual may require additional help learning to adapt periodically as new changes occur. But most individuals will get better quickly with a return to a protective environment.

Since RJ began treatment with Dr. Sen at the community psychiatry program, his behavior has steadily improved. This is due, in part, to a growing familiarity with his new surroundings, but it can also be attributed to better coping skills that his psychiatric treatment has provided him. RJ has begun to use words to describe his feelings and thoughts, which his therapist has facilitated and encouraged. With this increasing language use, RJ has had a significant decrease in the frequency and duration of his temper tantrums when he doesn't get his way.

Treatment begins with helping the patient, when possible (i.e., when the patient's ID is mild rather than moderate or severe), and the patient's family recognize who the patient *is*, at times using psychological testing, such as an IQ test or a personality inventory like the NEO-PI[3] (discussed in detail in part 2, case 3). Subsequently, the clinician, the patient (when possible), and the patient's family work together to set treatment goals related to this dimensional understanding of the patient's presentation. For example, *guiding* the patient and his family to recognize and adapt to, or, if possible, avoid, situations that provoke distress may be clinically relevant treatment goals. If such circumstances are unavoidable, guidance is provided about managing the distress in various ways. The psychotherapeutic process of guiding individuals with problems arising from a dimensional vulnerability is similar for individuals with ID and individuals with extremes of temperament. The difference is in the content of the therapy, which varies between these two groups and among individuals.

First, for the patient with ID, the clinician guides the patient (when possible) and his family to recognize how the patient differs from others along one or several dimensions of human psychological variance (whether from brain injury, genetic constitution, or experience). Next, the clinician helps them understand how this dispositional dimension renders the patient potentially vulnerable to certain life events provoking and sustaining an emotional response. It is useful to help the patient (when possible) and his family to see that the patient's response is one that all individuals can experience but—in him—can be excessive in degree or frequency. Perhaps most important, the clinician needs to help the patient (when possible) and his family appreciate his own contribution to his distress and—in all cases—help him manage it. For patients with mild ID, cognitive behavioral therapy can be especially helpful for enhancing recognition into their own contributions to their distress.

In contrast, a clinician treating a patient with a vulnerability of temperament works to strengthen the patient's resilience to provocation by teaching the patient to plan and practice responses and, if substance use is exacerbating the situation, helping the patient achieve and maintain abstinence. A patient can be *guided* to avoid or delay (awaiting a growth in maturity and judgment) certain provocations and to modify emotional responses via coaching or, in some cases, medication. Through these efforts, the clinician helps the patient alter contexts, modify maladaptive responses, and bring understanding. These goals are the same for individuals with vulnerable temperaments as they are for individuals with ID.

Summary Points

The dimensional perspective:

1 Focuses on individual psychological dimensions that are universal, measurable, and graded (cognition and temperament)

2 Has an underlying conceptual triad of *potential*, *provocation*, and *response*

3 Applies to psychiatric conditions that arise from who a person *is*

4 Suggests *guidance* as the treatment goal

CHAPTER FIVE

The Behavior Perspective

We addicts can always find one another. There must be some strange addict radar or something. . . . When he offered me that . . . well, my whole world pretty much changed after that. There was a feeling like—my God, this is what I've been missing my entire life. It completed me. I felt whole for the first time. . . . I guess I've pretty much spent the last four years chasing that first high. I wanted desperately to feel that wholeness again. It was like, I don't know, like everything else faded out. All my dreams, my hopes, ambitions, relationships—they all fell away . . .

—from Nic Sheff's *Tweak: Growing up on Methamphetamine*

The Case

Dr. Brown meets Ms. G, a 21-year-old pregnant woman, who presents to a perinatal substance abuse treatment program for help with her heroin addiction.

(Dr. Brown's comments are printed in *italics*.)

Hello, Ms. G, I'm Dr. Brown. I'd like to start by learning a little bit about your parents.

Well, I was adopted, so I don't know much about that part. My mother overdosed, and I don't know who my father is.

I'm so sorry to hear about your birth mother. What drugs did she use?

I know she used heroin because that's why she gave me up for adoption. She was 18 and too strung out to take care of me. They told me she used the whole time she was pregnant. I don't know anything about my father—I'm not even sure my mother knew who he was. She gave me up for adoption when I was just a few days old.

Where were you born?

In the Bronx, but I've been in Larchmont with my adoptive parents all my life.

Do you know anything about your birth history, like whether or not there were any complications with your birth?

I know I was premature and that I had withdrawal, but that's all I know. I don't want my baby to go through that. That's why I'm here.

We're glad you're here. How did you find us?

My dad's a doctor and he'd heard about the program before, so when I told them I was pregnant, they brought me here.

What does your mother do?

She's a lawyer.

How's your relationship with them?

Well, we used to get along great when I was little. It was just the three of us, you know, so we were pretty close. Then in high school I started running wild around the city and my parents still wanted to control my every move. And since then we've grown apart, but I know they're there for me.

(Ms. G is asked about and denies any problems during early childhood.)

How far did you get in school?

I made it to the twelfth grade but then dropped out when I'd missed too many days to graduate. It's a drag. . . . I was a straight A student until my last two years. Then my grades just tanked because I was never there. I want to get my GED, though, and go back to school.

What did you do after you left school?

I had a few jobs, but they never lasted more than a couple months. I was a cashier at a clothes store at my last job, but that was two years ago. I've basically just been tricking since then. I stopped doing that last year, too. That's when I started dancing.

Exotic dancing?

Yeah. It's rough, but it's better than being on the streets. I could only hide being pregnant for so long. They switched me to waiting tables after my first trimester. The money's not as good, but it's better than nothing, I guess.

How far along are you in your pregnancy?

I'm 30 weeks today.

Are you currently in a relationship with anyone?

I've been with my boyfriend since my junior year. He's locked up for drugs.

How old were you when you first had sexual intercourse?

17—with my boyfriend.

How many partners would you say you've had since that time?

You mean just for sex? 'Cause I've only had one boyfriend. I don't know; maybe fifty. That sounds pretty bad.

Do you use anything for birth control and to protect you from STDs?

Condoms. Mmm . . . sometimes.

Have you been pregnant before?

When I was 17, but I had an abortion early on.

(Ms. G is asked about and denies any sexual or physical abuse and any involvement with the criminal justice system.)

Is there any particular religion you believe in?

I was raised Catholic. I just started going back to church last week.

(Ms. G is asked about and denies any other mental and physical conditions [including HIV and hepatitis C], medications, and drug allergies.)

How would you describe yourself before you started using drugs?

I had a lot of friends and we were all pretty chill—it takes a lot to get me upset.

Were you a person who planned a lot or were you more impulsive?

Definitely impulsive—when I was with my friends, we'd come up with wild ideas all the time and just go do them. Some of them were pretty dangerous.

Such as?

Like once me and my friends got the idea of soaking tennis balls in gasoline cans. We lit the balls on fire and then played "fire tennis." It was crazy.

And now?

I'm just tired. I've been tired of using a long time now, but then when I found out I was pregnant, I knew I had to get off the drugs . . . all of them. I tried to do it on my own but it didn't work. I couldn't do it on my own. It was too hard.

Yeah, I imagine that can be pretty difficult to do. Well, I'm glad you decided to come in. What drugs were you using?

Weed, cocaine, heroin . . . I've tried them all. Heroin's what stuck, though. I fell in love.

So tell me about how your drug use started. Was marijuana first?

Yeah. I tried it first when I was away at camp after middle school. I don't smoke more than a blunt or two a month. I haven't had one in a few weeks . . . I just do it if it's around.

And the cocaine?

I tried that two summers later, when I was 16. This guy in the city turned me on to it. Back then I just snorted it that one summer. But, since then, I've shot it too, though not in a couple of months.

And the heroin?

That started during my junior year when I began seeing my boyfriend. He was using and wanted to turn me on to it. I was pretty much up for anything and, like I said, after that, it was love at first sight—with the heroin. Pretty soon I was shooting every day.

What about alcohol? How much do you drink?

That's not really my thing. It's doesn't do much for me. I haven't had a drink in a long time.

What about cigarettes, do you smoke?

I smoke about half a pack a day, but I didn't pick that up until I was 18.

So it sounds like you have been using marijuana, cocaine, and heroin fairly consistently for the past several years. Have there been any times when you've been able to quit?

About a year and a half after I started using heroin, my parents took me to a residential treatment program. I stayed there for fifteen months but as soon as I left I picked up the drugs again. I went to live with my boyfriend after leaving, so it was no surprise I started using again. I really hated myself for relapsing. Then my boyfriend got locked up and I moved back in with my mom and dad. When I found out I was pregnant, they helped me get in here. They're going to let me stay with them even after I have the baby. My boyfriend will probably be out of jail by then, but I don't want to live with him because I don't want to relapse.

That sounds like a good idea. And can you tell me how you're feeling now?

Pretty good. I've been eating better even though I've only gained 10 pounds. I'm sleeping better. I'm glad I'm getting help. I'm really looking forward to being a mom.

Sounds like you're feeling hopeful about the pregnancy and kicking this problem.

It's scary, but I know it's what I have to do. I am really excited about my church throwing me a baby shower in a couple of weeks. I feel like I have a lot of support and that makes me feel like things will work out.

MSE: Ms. G is a well-groomed, alert, and cooperative pregnant woman. She looks her stated age and maintains good eye contact throughout the interview. She demonstrates no tics or tremor. She is a good witness to her mental state and responds to questions without delay. Her speech is normal in rate, amount, and volume. It is not circumstantial and there is no evidence of thought disorder or aphasia. She describes her mood as great. She's excited about getting treatment and she appears euthymic. She has a full range of affect. She describes normal energy and motivation and normal concentration. She feels like she will be a good mother and is determined to remain drug free. She denies any thoughts of harming herself or the fetus. She has no hallucinations, delusions, obsessions, compulsions, or phobias. She is fully oriented and has a good fund of information, with an MMSE score of 30/30. Her intelligence is assessed to be above average, and her insight and judgment are normal.

The Discussion

Ms. G's case demonstrates concepts central to the behavior perspective. In this perspective, the underlying conceptual triad is *choice*, physiological *drive* (development of a "hunger" for the maladaptive behavior—such as use of a drug—that is experienced with the same powerful salience as everyday hunger for food, water, or sleep), and conditioned *learning* (maintenance of the behavior by the rules of conditioned learning).

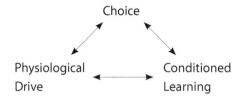

In essence, a behavior is something an individual *does*. Behaviors are *goal-directed* motor acts. Neurologists study what actions people can perform—such as walking, grasping, reaching, and running—and try to identify and explain disorders in these capacities. Psychiatrists, in contrast, study how people employ those capacities—how they *choose* to behave—and seek to identify and explain disorders in these choices. Behavioral disorders all involve goal-directed action but can be divided into three subgroups: disorders of innate drives (e.g., circadian sleep disorders, eating disorders, paraphilic sexual disorders), disorders involving acquired drives (e.g., substance use disorders, kleptomania, pathological gambling, pyromania), and disorders provoked by a social attitude resting on assumptions, overvalued ideas, or search for a role (e.g., conversion disorders, self-cutting, crime).

In this chapter a case of opioid dependence, an acquired drive disorder, is used to demonstrate the key features of the behavior perspective. An acquired drive, like an innate drive for food, can be felt in terms of a "hunger." Drive is a brain-based physiological process that influences and dominates the other cerebral faculties. Drive does this by producing an "attitude" that influences perceptions and decisions. For example, an individual who smells the aroma of a fresh-baked chocolate-chip cookie makes the decision to eat or not eat the cookie based on her attitude toward food at the time (whether she is in a state of hunger or satiety). However, drive and attitude alone do not determine behavior—we don't always eat a cookie when we're hungry nor are we always hungry when we choose to eat. The expression of drives is shaped by personal aspects of the individual—what she has *encountered,* who she *is* dimensionally, and any brain disease she might *have*. In this way, behaviors typically are shaped and can become increasingly adaptive or maladaptive, as Ms. G experienced with opioid use. In Ms. G's case, her brain's physiological reaction to heroin produced a "love at first sight" experience, which was the main reason she sustained the behavior. Also relevant to this case, however, are aspects of her life story (such as encountering a heroin-using boyfriend) and dimensional life (such as being of an impulsive temperament). In addition, as a cerebral faculty, drive can be deranged by structural or functional brain disease (such as certain genetic syndromes).

The study of behavior, its nature, its role, and its dynamics, was central to twentieth-century psychology. Sigmund Freud appreciated the importance of drive in psychological life but was unable to identify a biological structure in the brain that embodied drive. John B. Watson, considered the founder of behaviorism, documented how behavior can be shaped by learning, through rewards and punishments.[1] Building on the foundations of earlier scientists (and without addressing the underlying brain mechanisms), he stated that we learn to sustain behavior in three ways, via classical conditioning, operant conditioning, and social (observational) learning. Ivan Pavlov demonstrated via his series of classical conditioning experiments (pairing a dog's food to a bell's ring) that individuals are able to learn that one thing (a bell ring) leads to another (food).[2] B. F. Skinner's operant conditioning experiments, in which, for example, a lever press yielded rat food, showed that individuals can learn that one thing (a lever press) produces another (food).[3] Albert Bandura's work, in which an adult modeled to a child the behavior of hitting a doll, illustrated that individuals learn what to do (hit BoBo) from observing behaviors of a socially salient model (an adult).[4] Curt Richter drew together the ideas of Watson and Freud and advanced the field by identifying a biological brain structure that embodies a drive capable of being shaped by the environment (the suprachiasmatic nucleus regulates circadian cycles, and hence the drive for sleep, and is influenced by light via the optic nerve).[5] This line of research supports many conclusions about behaviors. It implies that genetically derived brain processes underlie certain behaviors and that these processes can be shaped by the environment. It demonstrates that people vary in how well these structures function and that individuals can differ in terms of homeostatic settings (e.g., some people need more food or less sleep). It also suggests that behaviors can be shaped by predispositions and consequences. The net result is that some behaviors may result from physiologic "overdrive" (as in Kluver-Bucy syndrome), maladaptive learning (as in a conversion disorder), or a combination of the two (as in substance use disorders).

In this case, Ms. G's genetic predisposition to opioid dependence seems apparent, given her birth mother's known opioid dependence. However, after adoption, Ms. G was raised in an environment where opioids were not readily available and opioid use was not a modeled behavior. It was not until Ms. G, in her teenage years, appropriately began to leave the protected environment of her parents' world that she encountered illicit drugs. Once introduced to these drugs by influential peers, she found she enjoyed marijuana, cocaine, and heroin, but she developed a particular hunger ("I fell in love") for heroin. In Ms. G we see the operational underpinnings of the behavior perspective. She has a genetically derived vulnerability to the euphoriant effects of opioids that went unexpressed in the absence of exposure to heroin. Once she made the choice to try heroin, she experienced the immediate and striking effects of the drug and learned to associate the two, thus acquiring a hunger for heroin and a drive to have it. Ms. G then continued to use heroin to again experience these effects. Thus, her opioid dependence illustrates the underlying conceptual triad of the behavior perspective: *choice,* physiological *drive* (development of a "hunger" for the maladaptive behavior that is experienced with the same salience as everyday hunger for food, water, or sleep), and conditioned *learning* (maintenance of the behavior by the rules of conditioned learning).

Ms. G's genetic predisposition to opioid dependence alone surely did not determine her initial use of opioids, although genes likely influenced her continued use. These genetic influences may have decreased the salience of parental and social efforts to dissuade her from drug use and increased the persuasive power of peers who provided her with the influence and opportunity to use. However, her behavior remained open to further influences. After she was persuaded to try heroin and after many months of regular use, she became pregnant. This event, along with parental support, persuaded her to enter substance abuse treatment with the goal of *interrupting* the behavior. Once in treatment, she received further external persuasion not to use and began to experience the rewards of abstinence. In this way, Ms. G has *learned to choose* not to use opioids. Her genes have influenced her behavior, but they are not determining her behavior: she has retained the freedom to make choices as an individual despite the influence of her genetic makeup on her initial response to heroin's euphoriant effects.

Although treating drug dependence can be challenging, with behavioral and pharmacologic treatments, Ms. G can be persuaded away from her drug use just as she was initially persuaded toward use. In drug-dependence disorders, the salience of positive consequences can be high, in that the drugs mimic biological reinforcements (for instance, many heroin users have compared the euphoria of their high to the experience of orgasmic release). In contrast to most other behaviors, an individual's experience of the positive effects of drugs is immediate, striking, and fairly reliable—and therefore powerfully effective for conditioned learning. This immediacy of positive experience is contrasted with the delayed effects of the negative experiences that accumulate with chronic drug use, such as withdrawal effects, incarceration, and loss of relationships. The role of choice is what defines the behavior perspective and is usually the center of any debate about the role of the individual in behavioral disorders. Although such a discussion is beyond the scope of this chapter, some of these issues will be discussed in part 2.

Summary Points

The behavior perspective:

1 Seeks to identify and explain disorders of individual choice

2 Has an underlying conceptual triad of *choice,* physiologic *drive,* and conditioned *learning*

3 Applies to psychiatric conditions characterized by what a person does

4 Suggests *interrupting* as the treatment goal

CHAPTER SIX

The Disease Perspective

"Tell me one last thing" said Harry, "Is this real? Or has this been happening inside my head?" Dumbledore beamed at him, and his voice sounded loud and strong in Harry's ears even though the bright mist was descending again, obscuring his figure. "Of course it is happening inside your head, Harry, but why on earth should that mean that it is not real?"

—from J. K. Rowling's *Harry Potter and the Deathly Hallows*

The Case

M r. L is a 60-year-old man who, four days after undergoing a lumbar laminectomy for chronic back pain, developed visual hallucinations for which a psychiatric consultation was requested. The psychiatrist, Dr. Milner, saw Mr. L on post-operative day five, in the presence of the patient's brother, who helped the patient recall some of the history.

(Dr. Milner's comments are printed in *italics*.)

Hello, Mr. L, I'm Dr. Milner. I'm a psychiatrist. Dr. S asked me to come and see you today. How are you feeling?

They've got me tied down here! How do you think I feel?

I imagine you're pretty upset. I talked to the nurses, and they said you were a bit confused and scared last night. That's why I'm here—to figure out what caused you to get so confused and scared so that I can help. You look awfully uncomfortable.

It's terrible. Tied up like a dog.

Yes, it is terrible, but Dr. S and the nurses were concerned for your safety.

I'm fine—I just want out of these and out of here.

Mr. L, I need to ask you a few questions as part of my evaluation.

Go ahead then.

First, has anyone in your family ever had any psychiatric conditions, like depression or schizophrenia?

My mother seemed pretty depressed most of her life, if you ask me, but she never took anything for it, except Librium. Both Mom and Dad have been gone a good while now.

(Mr. L's older brother added that one of their two sisters was successfully treated with fluoxetine for depression, but there is no other history of psychiatric conditions, including substance use disorder and suicide attempts, in the immediate or extended family.)

How did your parents die?

Mom had lymphoma and Dad had a stroke.

I'm sorry. Is your family from around here?

No, we're originally from St. Paul, Minnesota. I'm the only one who left. I've been here in Charlottesville since college. My brother's just here to help me with the surgery. It's just me at home, you know.

You live alone?

I'm a confirmed bachelor, I guess you'd say. I dated a woman once about fifteen years ago, but it only lasted for a few months. Seems she didn't love me as much as I loved her.

I'm sorry to hear that.

What's done is done. No use crying over spilled milk.

So you went to UVA?

Graduated there and then got my MBA from George Washington University.

What kind of work do you do?

I worked for the government from 1978 to 1997. I was a systems analyst. I'm retired now, but still do some consulting.

Do you smoke cigarettes?

Never.

What about alcohol?

I never was a big drinker—I can't stand the run-down feeling the next day. I drink a beer maybe once a week, at the most.

And any drugs?

Well, I smoked some pot in college, but never anything since.

And have you ever been arrested?

Well, I was pulled over for speeding when I was a teenager out in Minnesota. Not much to do out there when you're a kid. But, no, nothing else.

Are you religious?

We were raised Lutheran, but I don't go to church much.

How's your health, besides your back?

Other than that, nothing. But that's bad enough.

How long have you been having back trouble?

This has been with me, off and on, for over twenty years—that's when I had the first laminectomy. That went pretty well, but then I had my accident. That was seven or eight years ago. It was nothing serious, just a little fender bender, but it set me back. I had a discectomy and was okay again for a couple of years. Since then, the pain's come back and nothing can touch it. I've tried everything: steroids, physical therapy, even acupuncture.

So you had another laminectomy. How's your pain now?

It's completely gone. I was feeling back to normal, until I started seeing clouds.

Clouds?

Last night I just suddenly started seeing little clouds: they're just floating all around—all over the room—different colors and shapes. They're not as many right now—they sort of come and go as they please. When I reach out to touch one, my hand even feels wet. And the floor looks wet. They smell so sweet—like perfume—or lilies of the valley. And last night I also saw a little girl. She was standing right there in the corner and she looked like she was lost; she looked scared . . . so I got out of bed to try and help her, and that's when the nurses came in and put these on me. I've been awake most of the night watching out for her again.

And has she come back?

No. Not yet.

Are you hearing anything unusual or anything that other people can't hear?

No, right now it's just the clouds and the water on the floor. I know it's crazy, but they seem so real. I've never seen anything like this.

Any funny tastes?

No.

Were you taking any medications at home before you came into the hospital?

Just my pain medication—the hydromorphone—and I take a little diazepam so I can sleep through the pain.

How much is the diazepam dose?

Just 10 mg.

Have you ever experienced anything like this before?

No way. This is totally new.

Have you ever had any trouble with your mood at all? For example, any problems eating, feeling sad for days or weeks on end, trouble with your energy, thoughts of suicide?

Never. Not a bit. I think I'm one of the happiest people I know. If I get down, I never stay there for more than a day or two, you know; and then it's usually when the pain is getting the worst of me. But what's the point of being down about it, you know?

What about the opposite? Have you ever had a time when your mood was too good or your energy too high? Or a time when you didn't need sleep for days on end?

I wish I had more energy. Doesn't everyone? No, I've never been manic, if that's what you mean. Truth be told, I never thought I'd ever have a reason to see a shrink. This is a shocker to me.

(Upon review of the medical record, Dr. Milner found that the hydromorphone and diazepam were discontinued on admission to the hospital. Mr. L was started on morphine for pain control, which was tapered and discontinued by post-operative day four. At the time of the evaluation, he was receiving only a stool softener.)

MSE: Mr. L is a well-groomed and alert man lying in his hospital bed with both arms restrained. He is cooperative, but makes poor eye contact. He appears slightly restless. His speech is prompt and full without formal thought disorder. He describes his mood as "nervous" and looks slightly sad but is able to brighten at times.

He denies any change in his self-attitude and is hopeful for the future. He has no passive death wishes or suicidal or homicidal thoughts, plans, or intent. He describes visual, tactile, and olfactory hallucinations, but denies auditory and gustatory hallucinations. He denies any grandiose, persecutory, somatic, or other delusions. He denies obsessions, compulsions, or phobias. His MMSE score is 23/30. He misses 2 points on time orientation, 4 on attention/calculation, and 1 on recall.

The Discussion

Mr. L's case demonstrates concepts central to the disease perspective. In this perspective the underlying conceptual triad is *clinical syndrome, pathology* ("broken part"), and *etiology*.

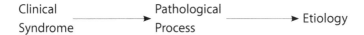

A disease is something an individual *has*; it comes on unbidden. The essence of the disease perspective is that brain structure and/or function is disrupted, resulting in psychiatric symptoms such as altered consciousness (as in delirium), decline in global cognition (as in dementia), or change in affect (as in bipolar mood disorder), executive/integrative function (as in schizophrenia), memory (as in Korsakoff syndrome), or language (as in the aphasias). In the case of Mr. L, he presented with a prominent change in level of consciousness. According to the nursing report, he appeared confused, restless, and frightened, attempting to get out of bed to rescue a girl that he alone could see.

The concepts of the disease perspective are standard in medicine and so are familiar to medical students and physicians. Clinicians are trained to recognize the clustering of signs, symptoms, and course that define a clinical syndrome. Clinicians then proceed to identify the bodily *pathology* generating the clinical *syndrome's* features, with the ultimate goal of finding the *etiology* (cause) of the *pathology* and, so, a *cure*. For instance, medical students, from their earliest clinical exposures to internal medicine patients, quickly learn to recognize the cluster of symptoms (e.g., shortness of breath, fatigue, swollen ankles, increased heart rate, lung crackles) that define the clinical syndrome of congestive heart failure

(CHF). As they proceed in their training, students—with the help of senior clinicians and a legacy of medical investigation—become increasingly able to discern from an array of possible structural or functional pathologies (e.g., myocardial infarction, mitral valve disease, hyperthyroidism) which is at play in an individual patient presenting with the *syndrome* of CHF. Identifying the *pathology* of CHF for a particular patient not only is relevant to *curing* that patient, but also may be helpful to the identification of the ultimate *etiology* of the *syndrome*. For example, it is now known that a patient who has CHF may have an inflammation of the pericardium (constrictive pericarditis), which can, in turn, be caused by a variety of etiologic factors. In immunocompromised patients, for example, an opportunistic *Staphylococcus aureus* infection may lead to constrictive pericarditis. Treating the patient for the bacterial infection may slow the progression of the pericardial disease and extend life. The same elements of the disease triad (*clinical syndrome, pathology,* and *etiology*) illustrated by CHF also apply to the clinical syndrome of dementia. Dementia, a disorder defined as a global decline in cognitive function occurring in clear consciousness, may be related to structural and functional pathological disruptions such as pernicious anemia and Huntington disease (HD), with their respective etiologies of vitamin B_{12} deficiency and triplet repeat genetic mutation (although we cannot link *etiology* to *pathology* to *syndrome* in HD as completely as we can link a bacterial infection to constrictive percarditis to CHF).

Using Mr. L's case, we will demonstrate how the elements of the disease triad link up. The first step is to define the clinical syndrome (signs, symptoms, and course) to answer the question: what is the nature and origin of the syndrome in which we suspect that brain function and/or structure has been disrupted? In the case of Mr. L, the symptoms include decline in cognitive function (manifested by confusion and lower-than-expected MMSE total score, given his educational and occupational history), altered level of consciousness (in this case hyperalertness as demonstrated by his restlessness and fear), and impaired attention (shown by the attention/calculation section of MMSE). In addition to these symptoms, Mr. L has abnormalities in his sleep-wake cycle (Mr. L reports being awake all night, which nursing confirmed, and his syndrome began at night), perception (visual, tactile, and olfactory hallucinations), mood (fear, sadness, and irritability), and behavior (getting out of bed against medical advice). The onset of these symptoms is acute and the course fluctuates, with worsening at night. The signs, symptoms, and course are typical of the syndrome known as delirium. Delirium usually takes one of two forms: a hypoalert or a hyperalert state (both characterized by a "clouding" of consciousness and difficulty focusing and sustaining attention).[1] In this case, Mr. L's communication with the examiner, Dr. Milner, occurs in a relatively lucid period and so is not impeded by inattention. However, interviewing such a patient is often challenging. Without such a careful history, a clinician can often confuse hyperalert delirium with a manic or schizophrenic episode. Although the core features of delirium are disturbances in cognition, consciousness, and attention, it is the abnormalities in mood and perception that are often most distressing to patients. The alterations in perception may occur in any sensory modality, but are most often—as seen with Mr. L—in the visual realm.

The second step required to link the elements of the disease triad is to tie the *pathology* in some way to the clinical *syndrome* using pathophysiologic reasoning. Delirium is a response of the brain to a variety of pathophysiologic processes and is not in itself an indication of a particular cause. Both the hypoalert and hyperalert forms may be associated with changes in electroencephalogram (EEG): generalized slowing and excess low-voltage fast activity, respectively. In both forms, the EEG abnormalities are proportional to the severity of the clinical presentation. In Mr. L's case, an EEG was not performed, as the diagnosis was easily made clinically. However, had an EEG been performed the night before Dr. Milner's evaluation, it most probably would have showed diffuse, excessive low-voltage fast activity, as is typical. With this suggestion of brain dysfunction, some might question whether Mr. L really has a psychiatric syndrome. Our response is to remind our readers, as Alois Alzheimer, a prominent psychiatrist at the turn of the twentieth century, believed,[2] that psychiatrists are interested in all disorders of thoughts, feelings, and behavior—regardless of their cause or origin. Delirium (also known as acute brain syndrome, encephalopathy, or intensive care unit [ICU] psychosis) is a syndrome whose core features of altered cognition, consciousness, and attention are also accompanied by abnormalities in perception, mood, and behavior. Delirium is a psychiatric syndrome that is an abnormal response of the brain to a pathophysiologic process affecting the brain.

The third step necessary in linking the elements of the disease triad, therefore, is improving knowledge regarding the *etiology* and pathogenesis of the *pathology*. Delirium is most commonly caused by metabolic disturbances, drug intoxication/withdrawal, infection, and hypoxia, often with several acting simultaneously. Of the metabolic etiologies, electrolyte abnormalities and organ failure are the most common. Drugs most likely to induce delirium include anticholinergics, narcotics, steroids, and antiparkinsonian agents. However, benzodiazepine, barbiturate, or alcohol intoxication can also cause delirium, as can withdrawal from these substances. Most of these precipitating causes tend to produce the hypoalert form of delirium. However, withdrawal from benzodiazepines, barbiturates, or alcohol is more likely to result in the hyperalert form. This form is more commonly known as delirium tremens (also known as DTs).

In the case of Mr. L, the acute onset of symptoms after several days of hospitalization, with no other identifiable cause, is a red flag for delirium tremens. The most important approach to treating a patient who has delirium is to identify the underlying cause, so as to effect a *cure*. If the underlying cause is intoxication, the syndrome will resolve with time; if the cause is metabolic, then the syndrome will resolve with correction of the metabolic abnormality. Dr. Milner recommended Mr. L take a one-time dose of diazepam 20 mg, followed by resumption of his usual 10 mg daily dose. Mr. L's delirium resolved within hours of his receiving the 20 mg dose and did not recur.

In contrast to the other common psychiatric conditions, such as dementia, bipolar disorder, and schizophrenia, delirium is a syndrome in which many of the components of the disease triad are often apparent.[3–5] Therefore, to most clearly elucidate the concepts of the disease triad, we chose to present a case of delirium here. Although the causal processes for these other psychiatric conditions are still unknown, clinical and research evidence suggests that a disruption of brain structure and function underlies all these conditions.[6–11] When elucidated, the etiologies for these conditions will most likely be more complex than those for delirium, as will the other components of the causal chain.

As seen with Mr. L's case, the disease perspective employs traditional medical reasoning to identify the *etiology* and *pathology* of a clinical *syndrome*. Just as dysfunction in motor and/or sensory brain regions/circuits leads to specific types of neurological syndromes, so dysfunction in specific brain regions/circuits leads to specific types of psychiatric clinical syndromes. Disease reasoning produces a testable model from which a clear line of progressive research can develop. It is the basis for the progress that has been made in medical research and holds great hope for the understanding and treatment of many, but not all, psychiatric conditions. Disease reasoning de-emphasizes the personal aspects of an individual's psychiatric condition and focuses on common features of the syndrome seen in other patients affected by it. For example, in this case, the personal details of Mr. L's life history and descriptions of his usual personality, although interesting and helpful to understanding him as a person, are less relevant to understanding the origin of his current symptoms than they would be in the case of a patient presenting with sadness immediately after the death of a spouse. More relevant is the stereotypic pattern of symptoms, such as visual hallucinations, and their course. Delirium is a syndrome seen among patients all over the world, with a range of life histories and personalities, who abruptly stop a benzodiazepine medication.

Summary Points

The disease perspective:

1 At its essence is about an abnormality in the structure or function of the brain expressed in the development of a syndrome
2 Has an underlying conceptual triad of clinical *syndrome, pathology,* and *etiology*
3 Applies to psychiatric conditions that a patient *has*
4 Suggests *curing* as the treatment goal

PART II

The Approach in Action

Introduction

Part 1 began by describing the foundation of the systematic psychiatric evaluation: a detailed history and MSE. The case-based
chapters in part 1 illuminate the key conceptual features of each of the
four perspectives of psychiatry, examining them one at a time. In part 2,
we apply these tools and concepts in a sequential way to a series of cases
with the goal of developing a formulation of and treatment plan for each
case. Most of these cases illustrate a presentation best understood from
one or two perspectives and are enhanced with commentary on the
remaining perspectives as they pertain to the case.

Step 1	Role induction
Step 2	History
Step 3	Mental status examination (MSE)
Step 4	Collateral information
Step 5	Consideration from each perspective in sequence
	• Life Story
	• Dimensional
	• Behavior
	• Disease
Step 6	Collaborative formulation
Step 7	Collaborative treatment plan

The box shows the step-wise approach to the systematic psychiatric
evaluation. We advise the reader to refer back to these steps while reading
the part 2 cases.

We begin each systematic psychiatric evaluation with a patient role
induction. In this brief step in the process we explain to the patient that
we do what any physician does, which is to take a history and do an
examination. By beginning with a role induction we ensure that every
patient has an accurate idea of what this evaluation experience will be

like. It's an important step because patients often have misconceptions about psychiatry and imagine the evaluation process as dissimilar from other medical specialties. By engaging the patient in the process, the physician has a better chance of winning the patient's cooperation, improving the validity of the history and MSE, and laying the groundwork for successful treatment. The patient knows that a lot of questions will be asked, but he or she also learns that there are confidentiality limits surrounding the answers given. By making clear that the formulation and treatment plan will be collaborative in nature and that questions can be asked, the doctor increases the chance of establishing an empathic rapport with the patient, who then becomes more likely to share history and inner experiences in an open and trusting manner.

In practice we begin each encounter with a role induction. However, since this is so similar from patient to patient, this step is demonstrated in part 2's first case only. All other steps appear in every case. As in part 1, every case in part 2 begins with a history (step 2) and MSE (step 3). In every case, we obtain collateral information (step 4). For every case, we systematically consider features of the presentation from each of the four perspectives (step 5), beginning with the life-story and followed by the dimensional, behavior, and disease perspectives. In examining each individual perspective, we ask which features can be explained by that perspective. For every case, we develop a formulation (step 6) and treatment plan (step 7) in collaboration with the patient and his or her family.

The importance of considering each case in this systematic and sequential way cannot be over-emphasized. In our experience, rushing to view a patient's psychiatric presentation from only one perspective to the neglect of others is one of the major pitfalls of psychiatric practice, one that contributes to untold patient and family suffering. Despite our combined forty plus years of clinical practice, we continue to consider each patient presentation from all four perspectives. As one gains experience in using the *Perspectives* approach, one may be able to synthesize and view the patients from all four perspectives simultaneously, but it remains essential to view each case from every perspective to gain a full understanding of the nature and origin of the patient's suffering and, thus, produce a complete formulation and treatment plan.

Bipolar Disorder

Maintaining Personhood in the Face of a Disease

Two days earlier, Ms. W, a 75-year-old woman, was admitted to the medicine service with chest pain, which was ultimately attributed to gastroesophageal reflux disease (GERD). While there, she was noted to have "behavior abnormalities," for which she was transferred to the psychiatry department, where she is now met by Dr. Postnikov.

(Dr. Postnikov's comments are printed in *italics*.)

Good morning, Ms. W, I'm Dr. Postnikov. How are you?

I'm very well today. And you, Doctor?

I'm fine, thank you. I'd like to start by learning more about you and what brought you here to the hospital.

I've been feeling quite fine, thank you; getting lots done. I haven't needed the least bit of sleep; I've been getting so much accomplished. My son—you know how children are—he worries about me so. He's the one who brought me here, but I've got a clean bill of health—tip-top. I'm ready to go home.

(Dr. Postnikov provides Ms. W the following role induction.)

I'm glad you're feeling so well. I'm going to be doing a standard psychiatric interview. There are a lot of questions, starting with your family history and then moving forward in time. You're welcome to stop me at any point to clarify and ask me questions, as well.

That's good to know. I'll be sure to ask if things are unclear.

After all my questions, I'll want you to tell me anything I didn't ask you that you think is important for me to know. Then we'll try to understand together what's been going on lately and how best to help you.

All right, dear, that sounds like a great way to proceed.

Everything you say to me will be entirely confidential, with just a few exceptions where I'm obligated to share information as needed to protect you and others—like if I learned that you were about to harm someone else or yourself—or if you were a victim of child abuse. Does all that sound okay?

Yes, dear, go right ahead. Fire away!

Can you tell me about your family, starting with your parents?

Mother was an avid gardener. Oh, how she loved to be outside. She would have loved this beautiful day. I miss her terribly this time of year. She died in her sleep at the grand old age of 80. Father had left us years earlier; he died of lymphoma, the dear. They were absolutely marvelous parents to us both. My brother's marvelous, although perhaps a bit too fond of the drink. And now I have three wonderful sons of my own—all boys. My youngest has depression, and I worry about him, of course, as any mother would.

Other than your son, has anyone else in your family been depressed or committed suicide?

Oh heavens, no.

(Ms. W is asked about and denies any problems during her gestation, infancy, and childhood.)

Can you tell me a bit about your education?

Oh, those were the best days of my life! I was top of my class at Miss Porter's and then off to Smith. I also took classes at Amherst and Oxford University. Education is very important to me!

Those sound like wonderful times. What kind of work did you end up doing when you left university?

I worked as a secretary for a U.S. senator and I loved being in the thick of things. I've worked my entire life—while raising my three boys I might add! I was something of an early feminist, but not a bra-burner, mind you! Since I've retired, I volunteer three days a week at my church library.

That sounds like a great way to spend your days. What kind of church do you belong to?

I come from a long line of Episcopalians, but I'm "multi-religional." You see, there is not just one true religion, so I try to read as much as I can about each religion. I attend the Quaker meeting near my home. But I always go back to the Episcopal Church: it's a glorious service. I love the organ and the hymns. (Ms. W starts singing.)

Ms. W, that's beautiful. You have a lovely voice. Is that your favorite?

Oh, I've got so many that I love. That was Mother's favorite. When I hear it, I think of her . . .

Ms. W, I'd like to change topic now and learn something about your marriage.

Charlie was a wonderful Amherst man! We had a whirlwind tour of Europe—Paris, Rome, Athens. We both loved to travel. We were married close to fifty years. He was my everything, my all, my soulmate.

It sounds like you had a wonderful marriage. When did he pass away?

He's been gone eight years now—lung cancer, the poor thing.

Ms. W, have you ever tried alcohol?

Charlie always took a drink every night. I made a perfect gin and tonic, if I must say so! I'd occasionally take one myself, but never more than one. Not good for the skin, you know.

And have you ever smoked cigarettes?

I tried smoking a few times—it looked so glamorous in the movies, you know—but Mother had a fit so that put an end to that.

Have you ever tried any illicit drugs?

Oh, heavens no!

I'd like to learn more about your medical history. Do you suffer from any chronic conditions?

Well, I've a bad heart, you know. I've already had one heart attack. They had to put one of those stents in there last year. My blood pressure and cholesterol are both sky high and my thyroid doesn't work too well either. Oh, the glories of old age.

Have you had any surgeries?

Just that heart stent business—that's when things started to go downhill for me. I was feeling perfectly fine until then, when all of a sudden I had chest pain and couldn't breathe. As it turns out, I was having a heart attack. Who would have thought?

Ms. W, how would you describe your personality?

I'm well bred but fiercely independent; just like Mother.

What do you enjoy doing for fun?

I'm a voracious reader. I abhor the television. I always played tennis growing up, but that's harder for me now. I still go walking every day, and swimming at my cousin's when the weather is fine. I've also started taking a ballet class—I love the dance. And I'm still involved in politics—I volunteer my time and give money to all the liberals. Did I tell you I'm a member of the NAACP?

No, that's fascinating. It sounds like you're leading a very active life. I'm glad for you. I'd like to ask you a bit about your past psychiatric treatment. Have you ever been hospitalized like this before?

Oh, so many times. The first time, that was back in the sixties, when I was a young mother, I was living in California and so excited about life. I didn't need to sleep for weeks. I was going full steam. But then I crashed and felt really down for about a year. And things just kept getting worse. I actually thought about ending it all. That's when my family really got worried and brought me to the hospital. It was a horrible experience. I was scared out of my mind. They made me get shock therapy, which they say worked, but I was terrified. The doctors diagnosed me with manic depressive illness and told me I should take a medicine—I think it started with an "L." I took that for several years and saw my psychiatrist, Dr. T, of whom I became quite fond. But eventually I felt so fine I let him go. And I found myself with even more energy and zest for life. I got so much accomplished in those days! My family and friends seemed alarmed, but I tell you, I've never been so productive! I didn't need to go back to the hospital because I was feeling just great. After Charlie died, I moved here, and I've stayed out of the hospital for the most part. Oh, my son took me in once after I first came out here because he said I was talking too fast, and in truth, I hadn't slept more than a few hours for several weeks. They brought me to the psychiatric floor and after my son told them all about my history, they told me I had bipolar disorder and prescribed valproic acid and another medicine to help me sleep, which was a marvelous help. It was the best I'd felt in a long time, when I was in there. They helped me a great deal. I'm eternally grateful for their kindness. I haven't had to see a psychiatrist in a long time though, since I found my geriatrician and alternative medicine doctor. They're both so brilliant and they take good care of me.

Ms. W, what brought you into the hospital this time?

I tell you, it all started eight months ago, when I had that darned stent put in. I keep feeling like I'm having another heart attack. Naturally, it's quite frightening, so I go to the emergency room. Two weeks ago this happened again but, when I went to the emergency room, they ran several tests and told me I didn't have a heart attack. They re-prescribed all of my medications, here is the list.

(Ms. W provides a list which indicates she was prescribed aspirin 325 mg po daily, lisinopril 5 mg po daily, nitroglycerin 0.4 mg SL prn chest pain, simvastatin 40 mg po hs, levothyroxine 50 mcg po daily, metoprolol 50 mg po daily, quetiapine 150 mg po daily, and valproic acid 500 mg po bid and 250 mg po hs.)

You know what? I'd never before taken the time to read all of the papers the pharmacist gives you! I spent the next two days reading all of them, and read about just the same side effects I was experiencing!

Such as?

Well, the papers said they cause fatigue and I had been feeling absolutely exhausted before I went to the hospital. I couldn't believe I was taking all of these medications and hadn't taken the time to read up on them! Naturally, I stopped taking all of the medications immediately, and ever since I've had so much more energy and am getting much more work done! I hardly need any sleep at all now! It feels great!

Thank you so much, Ms. W, for talking so much with me. It can be helpful to speak with someone in your family about your history, too. Is it okay with you if I call one of your family members and put them on speaker phone for the rest of the evaluation?

Oh of course. Call my son Jonathan.

(Dr. Postnikov calls Ms. W's eldest son, with Ms. W present and her son on speaker phone.)

Hello, Mr. W, my name is Dr. Postnikov. I've been talking with your mother, who is with me now. I wondered if you might be able to tell me about your mother's psychiatric history from your perspective.

Of course, thanks so much for calling. Mom has been sick with bipolar disorder since her mid-20s. She was in and out of psychiatric hospitals for most of my childhood. There are times when she's just fine, especially when she takes her lithium, but those don't last more than a year at most. And, even then, she's a pretty intense person—very passionate and in the moment. But then when she gets manic like this, she usually needs to be hospitalized. She's almost never been depressed and usually comes out of those times without any trouble. Three years ago, my wife and I convinced her to move from California to assisted living here to be closer to us and to be around people her own age. She's been doing much better since she's been here. She has a geriatrician and a family practitioner who specializes in alternative medicine. The family doc encourages Mom to take a bunch of stuff: a multivitamin, vitamin C, iron, calcium, vitamin D, you name it. He says he can cure her bipolar disorder. She likes her doctors, and it's great that she's only been in the hospital once in the last three years, but we really think she needs to have a psychiatrist.

Thanks for that information. Your mother tells me she's led a very exciting life, going to Smith, Amherst and Oxford, touring Europe, working for a senator . . .

Yes, believe it or not, that's all true. Mom's quite an accomplished woman. She's always been adventurous and enjoyed being where the action is.

Thank you, this is very helpful. Mr. W, what have you been noticing that made you want to bring your mother in to the hospital this time?

Well, first off, for the last week or so, Mom's mood has been very up; she's been talking so much it's hard to get a word in edgewise. She told me she stopped taking all of her medicines because they were making her feel tired. She said she was reading more than five different books at once and sleeping only a couple of hours a night. She pawned her jewelry and went on one big shopping spree: she bought twenty different Hermès scarves. I got so worried that I called her doctors. The family doc called Mom and even he was shocked at how fast she was talking. He told her to go back on all of her medications. But, unfortunately, she refused. I felt I had no choice but to bring her to the emergency room for her own good. They admitted her to make sure she wasn't having a heart attack, and she wore them out with her talking! They called the psychiatrist, who got her transferred over to psychiatry. We're just happy she agreed to be transferred.

MSE: Ms. W is a petite woman wearing multiple layers of clothing, including a hospital gown and a long suede trench coat, along with socks, ballet slippers, and a red hat. She walks with a cane, with her head held high. She exhibits no restlessness or tremor. She does not appear to be responding to any external stimuli. She appears distracted during the interview, although she makes good eye contact. Her speech displays increased rate, a syncopated rhythm, and loud volume, although there is appropriate articulation. Her speech is both tangential and circumstantial but is not marked by flight of ideas or loosening of associations. She describes her mood as "feeling fine," but she appears euphoric and expansive. Self-attitude and vital sense are both elevated. She adamantly denies suicidal and homicidal ideation. She denies any auditory, visual, olfactory, gustatory, and tactile hallucinations. When asked whether she has any special powers or is on a special mission, she replies that she is "obtaining top secret clearance by the CIA for government work abroad." She refuses to elaborate on this. She denies any persecutory delusions. She denies obsessions, compulsions, and phobias or other anxiety symptoms. Her intelligence is judged to be above average, she has an excellent fund of knowledge and is able to reason abstractly. Her MMSE score is 27/30, missing 3 on serial subtractions. Her insight into her mental illness and judgment on admission are fair.

The Discussion

Step 1: Role Induction

As with every case, we begin the psychiatric interview with role induction. Dr. Postnikov prepares Ms. W for the systematic nature of the interview, including the fact that a lot of questions will be asked of her and that there are confidentiality limits surrounding her answers. Dr. Postnikov also lets Ms. W know that the formulation and treatment plan will be collaborative in nature, and that she is welcome to elaborate on questions asked, ask questions of Dr. Postnikov, and offer any observations that she thinks are relevant to Dr. Postnikov's understanding of her case. In so doing, Dr. Postnikov increases the chance of establishing an empathic rapport with Ms. W, who then becomes more likely to share her history and inner experiences in an open and trusting manner with Dr. Postnikov. Thus, the psychiatric history and MSE conducted by Dr. Postnikov with Ms. W, and augmented with collateral information from Ms. W's son, serves as a valid point of reference for understanding and treating her.

Steps 2–4: History, MSE, and Collateral Information

In Ms. W's case, as in all cases, the psychiatric interview will serve as the point of reference for the formulation of the case and development of the treatment plan, and so we begin our discussion with a review and summary of Ms. W's history, MSE, and information from collateral informants, in this case Ms. W's son.

Ms. W and her son describe a long history of an episodic illness, which is usually well controlled with lithium carbonate treatment. However, about two weeks prior to admission, Ms. W stopped this medication and the symptoms of the illness quickly returned. These symptoms include euphoric mood, decreasing need for sleep, increased energy and motivation, difficulty concentrating, expansive view of herself and her future, poor financial decision-making, and grandiose delusions. As with prior episodes, Ms. W's cognition is intact during this episode, and the illness is occurring in clear consciousness.

Ms. W is usually an outgoing and active woman who is proud of her upbringing, education, and many achievements. In the past eight years, Ms. W has suffered two major stressors in her personal life: the death of her husband eight years ago, with which she coped well, and a myocardial infarction (MI) requiring stent placement eight months ago. Since having the stent placed, Ms. W has been more anxious about her physical health, prompting several emergency room visits to rule out an MI.

Step 5: Consideration from Each Perspective

The Life-Story Perspective

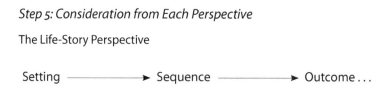

For this first case in part 2, we are repeating details from the history to demonstrate how historical details are necessary to consider a case from the life-story perspective. However, not all of the history details will be repeated in the life-story sections in subsequent cases. Instead, the reader is advised to refer back to the case history.

Ms. W's current difficulties have occurred in the setting of an MI and stent placement eight months prior. Anxiety about her cardiac health, coupled with GERD-induced chest pain for the past eight weeks, has prompted Ms. W to visit the ED several times during this period. However, the existing symptoms have been present for less than two weeks, coincident with her decision to stop taking lithium carbonate. It was in this context that she developed markedly increased energy, an elated mood, imprudent spending, and—most importantly—a grandiose delusion. These signs and symptoms are those of a lifelong illness that cannot be understood as arising in a meaningful way from concerns about her heart condition. Ms. W does not always take the lithium carbonate as prescribed, in part because she believes it causes her to feel fatigued. However, she also does not fully appreciate that her treatment with lithium is essential, or the likely risk of relapse when she stops taking it. Although we can empathically understand that she stopped taking lithium carbonate, and all her other medications, because she believed that they were making her tired, we cannot empathically understand the outcome of that decision, which was not a return to her baseline level of energy, but the recurrence of her illness. In this case, life-story reasoning can help explain the lack of insight into her illness and nonadherence to a medication regimen, but it seems inadequate to account fully for the origin of Ms. W's psychiatric condition.

The Dimensional Perspective

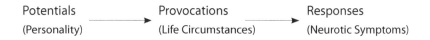

In chapter 5, we introduced the concepts of the dimensional perspective as they relate to intelligence via a case of intellectual disability. In part 2's case 3, we will discuss the concepts of this perspective as they relate to temperament. Therefore, for this case, we will limit our discussion to Ms. W's intelligence. Throughout her life, Ms. W has been a very smart woman. Although she presents with psychiatric symptoms that are not consistent with her usual attitude and behavior, the symptoms do not appear to have their origin in where she rests on the intelligence dimension. Therefore, for the purposes of this case, we can conclude that Ms. W's present condition is not arising from who she is intellectually and so is not best understood by the dimensional perspective.

The Behavior Perspective

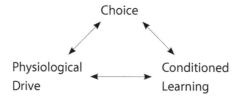

As always, we are trying to understand a patient's present illness in the context of her past psychiatric history. If a patient has been engaging in a pattern of repetitive innate or acquired behaviors to achieve a certain end, then her present condition may be explained, in part or wholly, by this perspective. In Ms. W's case, she is engaging in a pattern of behaviors, but they are not allowing her to achieve a certain end (i.e., they are not goal-oriented). Ms. W's repetitive behaviors do not appear to be relevant to the origin of Ms. W's current presentation.

The Disease Perspective

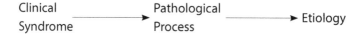

Disease-reasoning begins with the identification of a syndrome, so the first thing we want to know is whether Ms. W's illness has the form of a syndrome: a cluster of symptoms that occur together, run a course together, and respond to treatment together. (This statement is true for every case that follows but is not repeated in the disease section of the discussion of each case.) Ms. W's illness clearly has that form—one that has been described across cultures and across centuries (though it has been given various names). And although with bipolar disorder, as with other psychiatric conditions for which disease-reasoning may be appropriate, we have only hints of clinicopathological correlations (e.g., the fact that identical syndromes occur in the setting of damage to certain parts of the brain, the fact that the idiopathic syndrome is associated with certain abnormalities in brain function or structure) and only hints about etiology (e.g., from the results of genetic studies), based on what we know to date, disease-reasoning seems appropriate to explain Ms. W's illness. In a psychiatric condition best explained by the disease perspective, we expect there to be a "broken part," an *abnormality in the structure or function of the brain.*

In a patient who has mania we can't demonstrate an abnormality that is corrected by lithium (unlike the situation with, for example, diabetes, where we can demonstrate that the fasting blood sugar level [a proven reflection of pancreatic function] is corrected by insulin). However, we can note Ms. W's precipitous onset of psychotic manic symptoms after stopping lithium carbonate. This, coupled with her long history of stereotypic episodes of depressive and manic symptoms in the absence of treatment, suggests a disease of the brain as an explanation for Ms. W's current presentation.

Steps 6 and 7: Formulation and Treatment Plan

Ms. W's case does not present a diagnostic dilemma. The psychiatric signs are noticeable from across the room, and she describes a wealth of symptoms. She suffers from an episodic illness with characteristic changes in mood (elation, less frequently depression) accompanied by changes in self-attitude, energy, sleep, and libido. She carries herself in an oddly regal way and is bizarrely dressed. She appears overly full of vim and vigor, and her pressured and mildly thought-disordered speech and euphoric mood become evident rapidly during the evaluation. In addition, she clearly has delusions of grandeur. We conclude that Ms. W's current condition is best understood as something she *has*, rather than arising from something she has *encountered*, who she *is*, or what she is *doing*. Ms. W has the disease bipolar disorder for which the pathologic etiology and mechanism are as yet unknown. A resumption of lithium carbonate would be the recommended pharmacologic treatment. We include her case here not to offer a complex case for formulation, but for other reasons.

First, we want to emphasize the benefit of beginning with the life-story perspective even when there is little doubt as to the disease origin of the illness. Beginners in psychiatry are sometimes overly confident in giving their diagnostic impressions. Applying the perspectives in a systematic sequence protects against the tendency to mistakenly rush to a disease explanation for a patient's illness—an approach that even more experienced psychiatrists have been known to take. Given Ms. W's history of bipolar disorder and current symptoms of mania, we agree that her present illness is unlikely to be a direct result of personal life events, but the life-story perspective is relevant nevertheless. The timing of the current episode may, in part, be related to the stress of the recent cardiac procedure. Ms. W's lack of insight into the recurrent nature of the illness and the beneficial effects of lithium carbonate treatment, and her nonadherence to lithium, are other life-story factors relevant to the current presentation. Even in a syndromic presentation like Ms. W's, it is always important to consider first the patient's condition from the life-story perspective. It helps us remember that even when there is a disease to be treated, there is still a patient who needs our care. Ms. W's case demonstrates how taking a thorough and detailed history and then considering the patient from the life-story perspective—two key elements of the *Perspectives* approach—enables the clinician to connect empathically with the patient and to view her as more than a diagnostic label.

As part of residency training at Johns Hopkins, we were required to read a book by the founder of the American mental hygiene movement, Clifford Beers. He, and all of his four siblings, had symptoms of bipolar disorder, for which all five required hospitalizations. It was Beers's experiences in private and state psychiatric hospitals, including being subjected to deplorable conditions and severe maltreatment, that prompted him to write his 1908 memoir describing his illness and documenting the inhumane treatment he received.[1] With the help of William James, the memoir got the attention and support of the medical community—including that of Adolf Meyer—enabling Beers to champion reforms in the treatment of patients with psychiatric conditions. Beers founded the first outpatient psychiatric program in the United States, and it was his memoir that prompted Henry Phipps to fund the building of the first general hospital–based psychiatric unit, at the Johns Hopkins Hospital.

We recommend Beers's memoir to our students, as well as to readers of this book. Studying his story enables us to appreciate from the patient's point of view the experience of being in a psychotic state and the consequences for a person who needs humane care but does not receive it. This recommendation comes from our desire to ensure that future generations of psychiatrists and other clinicians remember that psychiatric conditions, including diseases like bipolar disorder and schizophrenia, occur in the context of a life, a family, and a community. Although the nature of her disease is clear, Ms. W is much more than that disease. As Ms. W tells her story, she is constantly reminding us of this. She was a college student and a wife. She is a mother. She is still full of life. She has a story to tell, as do all of our patients, if only we will listen—as the *Perspectives* approach, which begins with taking a detailed life history, enabled Dr. Postnikov to do with Ms. W.

Case Conclusion

Ms. W is wary of restarting her medications. During her hospitalization, the treatment team, including Ms. W's trusted geriatrician and alternative medicine doctor, explores and addresses further the medication side effects that are of most concern to Ms. W. Eventually, Ms. W decides to resume her home medications (including lithium carbonate). Subsequently her mood stabilizes, and she is discharged home with follow-up at a geriatric psychiatry day program. Prior to discharge, the following conversation takes place:

> *How do you feel about your stay here in the hospital and your illness, Ms. W?*
>
> I know I have bipolar disorder, and have had it most of my life. But I'm a romantic at heart and I think I'm in good company. I know many accomplished people who have had this illness—scientists, artists, musicians, and even doctors like you. The illness has given me the energy to explore many interesting things and provided me curiosity and strength. If given the choice to live without manic depressive illness, I would decline, as it has added to my life in so many ways—although I know that my family, who have been through hell with me and this illness, may disagree.

Summary Points

1 Role induction is an important first step in every psychiatric evaluation

2 It is always important to begin with the life-story perspective, even when there is little doubt as to the disease origin of the patient's illness

3 Even when there is a disease to be treated, there is still a person who needs our care

A Young Man with Psychosis

The Role of Life Story and Behavior in Disease

M r. N, a 22-year-old man, is admitted from the ED to the psychiatric unit after hearing a voice telling him to jump off the roof. Mr. N allows Dr. Chatterjee to call his outpatient psychiatrist but declines to give him permission to speak to any member of his family. Mr. N reluctantly agrees to the interview with Dr. Chatterjee. After several days, Mr. N allows Dr. Chatterjee to contact his father, but no other members of his family.

(Dr. Chatterjee's comments are printed in *italics*.)

Hi, Mr. N, why don't we start with you telling me about your family? Is your father still alive?

. . . Yes . . .

I'm glad to hear that. Does he live with you?

. . . No . . .

Where does he live?

. . . In Minnesota . . . You won't be able to talk to him there . . .

Why won't I be able to talk to him?

(A long silence passes and Mr. N does not answer the question.)

Minnesota is pretty far away from us here in Delaware. Do you get to see him often?

. . . No . . .

And your mother, where does she live?

. . . At home . . .

Where is home? Do you live with your mother?

. . . Only when I'm at home . . .

(At this point in the interview, Mr. N becomes mute and is unable to answer additional questions about his mother. Dr. Chatterjee later learns from Mr. N's father [who has no psychiatric history] that when Mr. N's mother was in her early thirties she had her only psychiatric hospitalization for a "nervous breakdown." Mr. N was 14 years old at the time. Since then, Mr. N's mother has continued to suffer from depression and anxiety but has refused further treatment. Mr. N's parents separated when Mr. N was 16 years old.)

> *Mr. N, I know your sister brought you to the Emergency Department. Do you have any other brothers or sisters?*

(Mr. N does not respond to the question. Instead, he appears to look past Dr. Chatterjee with his eyes affixed to something in the corner of the room. Mr. N smiles, and then laughs.)

> *Mr. N, did something funny make you laugh?*

(Instead of answering the question, Mr. N stands up, turns around, and walks away from Dr. Chatterjee. Dr. Chatterjee concludes the interview, reviews Mr. N's medical record, and contacts Mr. N's outpatient psychiatrist from whom Dr. Chatterjee learns that Mr. N was admitted to another hospital six months earlier when he experienced auditory hallucinations commanding him to drink liquid dishwasher detergent, for which he was treated surgically and then medically before transfer to the hospital's psychiatric unit. During that hospitalization, Mr. N was diagnosed with schizophrenia. Mr. N was treated with haloperidol and supportive psychotherapy and, two months later, when the hallucinations greatly diminished, he was discharged to an outpatient psychiatrist for continued treatment. His outpatient psychiatrist has seen Mr. N once only, a week after discharge from the hospital. Mr. N has missed all subsequent appointments with her and presumably has been on no medication for approximately three months. Dr. Chatterjee decides to reinitiate Mr. N's haloperidol treatment. Over the next five days, Mr. N gradually improves and Dr. Chatterjee is able to resume Mr. N's formal psychiatric evaluation.)

> *I'm glad that you're feeling well enough to be able to sit down with me today to have a conversation. I'd like to pick up our interview where we left off last time. I had asked you a little bit about your family. Would it be all right if we pick up from there?*

(Mr. N nods slowly but remains silent.)

> *OK, great. I understand you have an older sister. How old is she?*

28. She works for a lawyer.

And tell me a little about your brother. How old is he?

24 years. He's in college.

(Mr. N is asked about the mental and physical health of his siblings and extended family members and denies any problems except in his maternal uncle, who lives in Egypt and has been diagnosed with schizophrenia.)

I understand you were born in Egypt?

Yes, Cairo.

And your birthday is in February, I see.

February 15.

How long did you live in Egypt before you moved to the United States?

We left to go to Canada when I was 10. When I was 14 we moved here.

(Mr. N is asked about and denies any problems during gestation, infancy, and childhood.)

How old were you when you finished high school?

18. I started out with all As, but I wasn't that good a student at the end.

What have you done since you graduated?

I did some landscaping jobs during the summer, but I don't work anywhere now. I've been looking, but I can't find anything.

Any plans to go to college?

No.

I understand right now you're living at home with your mother and brother?

That's right.

And what kinds of things do you do to occupy your time?

I read the Bible. On Sundays we all go to church. We're Christian—they call us Coptics.

I see, and do you do anything else? Do you have a girlfriend or boyfriend?

No.

When is the last time you had a significant relationship with someone?

I had a girlfriend in high school, but she went off to college.

Are you currently sexually active?

No. Only with her.

Shifting gears a bit, do you smoke cigarettes?

Yeah.

When did you start smoking?

... 14 or 15.

How much do you smoke now?

Half a pack a day.

Do you drink alcohol?

I used to drink a half pint of vodka every day, but I haven't been able to drink since all this happened.

When were you drinking a half pint a day?

After I graduated; I thought maybe it would help the voices. I tried it for about two months, but no luck.

Have you ever smoked marijuana?

Yes. I started that when I moved here.

So you were about 14; how often were you smoking it then?

Every day.

Have you ever quit, or are you still using it?

I still smoke weed, just not as much.

How often do you use it now?

Maybe once or twice a week, but only if it's around.

What does smoking do for you?

I don't know anymore. When I first smoked I was new and didn't know anybody. I was just trying to make friends and they had some, so I smoked it. I really wasn't that into it at first, it wasn't like me. But then, when the voices started up, it seemed to chill them out—the voices. But now, I don't know, weed doesn't seem to do much for me anymore. Now, I smoke 'cause there's nothing else to do.

(Mr. N denies using any other illicit drugs, and his urine toxicology screen on admission is positive only for cannabinoids.)

Let's talk about your medical conditions. From looking at your record, I see that you were hospitalized for quite some time about six months ago. What happened?

I drank detergent and it exploded my esophagus. They had to do a surgery to fix it. But now I can't swallow and have to eat through this (gestures to his gastric tube). They tried to open up my esophagus more, but it hasn't worked yet. I want to be able to eat again, though.

(Mr. N denies any other medical conditions or surgeries, medications, and drug allergies.)

Do you remember Dr. L, your outpatient psychiatrist?

Oh, yeah. I liked her. But she's too far away.

Do you go to any other doctors?

No.

(Dr. Chatterjee conducts a medical review of systems. Mr. N answers "No" to each question except the following:)

And you're still having difficulties swallowing?

Yes, that's been the same ever since I drank that stuff.

I'm sorry to hear that you're still having trouble with that. I know that must be hard to deal with. On top of everything, I understand that you're still hearing voices. Tell me, when did this first occur? You said they started up after you began smoking marijuana?

Yeah. I guess it started when I was around 15. . . . They were just mumbles then, very quiet. At first I could just ignore them.

What was it like when you first experienced that?

I was just sitting in my room, chilling out, and I heard somebody whispering to me. It freaked me out, 'cause I thought someone was punking on me. You know, trying to trip me out. But no one was there. After that, it wasn't all the time, like it is now. . . . Back then I couldn't make out what they said. . . . They were quiet enough that I could distract myself from them. Then about a year ago they started getting louder . . . and a lot clearer. When I first heard the whispering, it was scary. It was like all "Friday the 13th" or something. It was like somebody's crept up behind me, whispering at me. I would turn around, and no one was there. Then I learned not to look every time and sort of got used to them. But now, they're so loud I can't ignore them.

What do you think is causing them?

. . . I know this sounds crazy, but I think it's a super power I have, like the voices are spirits and I'm communicating with people from the past and the future. It's also like déjà vu a lot. Sometimes when I meet new people I feel like I've met them before in a past life or something.

How many different voices do you often hear?

I've heard lots of voices before . . . maybe five or six, but now it's mainly just two of them. One is like an evil voice, and the other is a good voice. Sometimes I think the evil voice is of Hosni Mubarak and the good voice is Obama. But I'm not sure. They tell me to do all sorts of little things, like pick up that book off the table, or go down the hall and walk into that room. Stupid stuff.

What happens if you don't do what they say?

They'll keep talking about me, saying, "There he goes; he's walking down the hall. He's picking up that pencil off the table."

How are you able to hear their voices when they are physically hundreds of miles away from you?

. . . I guess that's part of my power.

Do you feel like you're receiving a direct signal from them or a message that is broadcast to you directly?

It's like when I hear them telling me to pick up the book, then the thought comes into my head that I should pick up the book.

When that occurs, do you feel like it is your own thought to pick up the book, or does it feel like it's someone else's outside thought that you should pick up the book?

It's an outside thought, and that's why I do it when sometimes I don't want to.

Do you feel as if you can resist those thoughts sometimes?

Yes. It's hard sometimes, though, when the voices are very loud. It gets too much for me to handle.

Mr. N, I'd like to talk more now about your past hospitalization when you were here a few months ago. Tell me about the injury that happened to your esophagus. Why did you drink the detergent?

The voices told me to drink it. They told me that I wouldn't die and that I had to do it.

From reading your medical record it appears that you had a pretty bad injury. Your esophagus ruptured, and you were hospitalized in the Surgical Intensive Care Unit.

I still can't eat, because when I swallow, the food gets caught. That's why I still have this (indicates feeding tube).

So, how do you get enough nutrition every day?

I squirt three protein shakes down the tube: breakfast, lunch, and dinner.

Does anyone help you with getting the shakes down the tube when you're home? Does anyone help you with cleaning it?

No. I can do it all myself.

Good for you! Looking back at your medical record, it appears that you've lost about 20 pounds since you were first hospitalized. You're a very thin guy. We're afraid that you haven't been getting enough food. Would it be okay if our nutritionist came by to talk to you about that?

Yes.

From your records, it appears that Dr. C performed your esopha-geal repair. Did you ever go back to see him?

No, I missed that appointment too, but I need to see him. I really want to be able to eat again.

Sure, we can help you with that. It must be pretty awful not to be able to eat. And feeding yourself through a tube sounds like a lot of work. The next thing I'd like to talk about is what brought you to the hospital this time. What happened?

I got scared and told my sister I wanted to come here. The voices were getting loud again. They told me to jump out the window. I went up to the third story in our house and walked over to the window, but I didn't want to do it. That's when I told my sister.

I know that when you left here last time, they had prescribed you a medicine called haloperidol. Did that medication help with the voices?

I think so, but I thought I could deal with the voices by myself. I mean, they've been with me for years. It's only lately they've been giving me real trouble.

I understand, but I think it's important that you keep on your medications. Has anyone told you before that they thought you had a disease called schizophrenia?

Yes.

What does it mean to you when people say that you have schizo-phrenia?

. . . I don't know.

MSE: Mr. N is a well-groomed young man wearing jeans and a tee shirt. His movements are slowed and he exhibits arm and leg restlessness. He does not exhibit tremor. He makes good eye contact, at times of piercing quality. His speech displays decreased rate, monotonous tone, normal rhythm, and soft volume. Articulation is appropriate. His speech is not marked by flight of ideas or loosening of associations. Mr. N describes his mood as "okay," and appears euthymic, but blunted. Vital sense is poor, but self-attitude is good. Mr. N describes a passive death wish, but denies any suicidal and homicidal ideation. He describes auditory hallucinations but denies visual, olfactory, gustatory, and tactile hallucinations. Mr. N describes persecutory delusions, in addition to thought broadcasting, thought insertion, and a belief that he can time-travel. He denies obsessions, compulsions, and phobias or other anxiety symptoms. His intelligence is judged to be above average. He has a good fund of knowledge and is able to reason abstractly. His MMSE score is 28/30, missing the date and floor of the building. Mr. N's insight into his mental illness and judgment are poor and fair, respectively.

The Discussion

Step 1: Role Induction

We have omitted or abridged the presentation of role induction for this case and the cases that follow, but we want to emphasize that we conduct the step of role induction in the evaluation process with every patient.

Steps 2–4: History, MSE, and Collateral Information

Mr. N was born in Egypt, emigrated to Canada at age 10, and came to the United States at age 14. He was quiet and shy with no behavior problems while growing up in Egypt and Canada. After the family moved to the United States, Mr. N's mother began struggling with untreated depression and anxiety. It was around this time that Mr. N began smoking cigarettes and marijuana daily. When Mr. N was 16 his parents separated and his father moved from Delaware to Minnesota. After that, Mr. N had little contact with his father. At age 21, Mr. N began drinking heavily, which lasted for a period of two months. Mr. N continues to smoke marijuana, now approximately twice weekly.

Mr. N has a seven-year history of a psychiatric condition, in the setting of regular marijuana use. Initially this illness was marked primarily by auditory hallucinations. In the past year these hallucinations increased in volume and clarity and became increasingly distressing. Six months ago Mr. N ingested dishwasher detergent in response to command auditory hallucinations. Because of the resultant esophageal erosion, Mr. N required surgical and medical intervention. Mr. N was seen by the consultation-liaison psychiatrist who diagnosed schizophrenia and recommended treatment with haloperidol. He was then transferred to the inpatient psychiatric unit where his medication treatment continued and behavioral therapies began. After four weeks on the psychiatric unit and two months in the hospital, Mr. N's auditory hallucinations lessened, but his other symptoms (e.g., social withdrawal, formal thought disorder, thought blocking, blunted affect, and grandiose delusions) showed little response to treatment. Mr. N was discharged from the hospital and referred to Dr. L for continued medication and behavioral treatment as an outpatient. Mr. N kept only his initial intake appointment with Dr. L and continued to smoke marijuana once or twice a week.

Three months or more prior to the present admission, Mr. N stopped his antipsychotic medication. Two weeks prior to admission, he began behaving strangely. The hallucinations, this time commanding him to jump out the window, returned. Mr. N told his sister, who brought him to the ED for evaluation. On admission, Mr. N's cognition was intact and his symptoms were occurring in clear consciousness.

Of note, although Mr. N initially declined Dr. Chatterjee's request to contact any member of his family, Dr. Chatterjee eventually won enough of Mr. N's trust to get permission to speak with his father, which improved the validity of the interview as a point of reference for formulating Mr. N's case and developing his treatment plan.

Step 5: Consideration from Each Perspective

The Life-Story Perspective

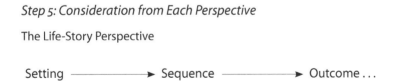

Mr. N's symptoms include formal thought disorder, apathy, social withdrawal, blunted affect, grandiose delusions, and command and commenting auditory hallucinations. These cannot be understood as arising in a meaningful way from his immigration to the United States, his mother's illness, his parents' separation, or his current stressors. Nevertheless, these are all significant events in Mr. N's life that preceded either the initial onset or relapse of his symptoms. Psychiatric symptoms are more prevalent in immigrants and children with a psychiatrically ill parent, and are more likely to occur after major stressors such as moving, a parent's illness, or parents' separation (if stormy). And, of course, worsening or return of symptoms is more likely to occur in the presence of ongoing stressors, such as inability to feed by mouth. In this case, life-story reasoning may help explain the precipitation of Mr. N's illness, the time of its onset, its sustained nature, and even the recent relapse. However, life-story reasoning seems inadequate to account fully for the nature, origin, and symptoms of Mr. N's psychiatric condition. One might expect sadness, or demoralization, after such a sequence of events, but not grandiose delusions or command auditory hallucinations.

The Dimensional Perspective

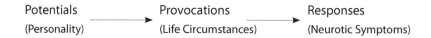

Potentials (Personality) → Provocations (Life Circumstances) → Responses (Neurotic Symptoms)

For the purposes of this case, we will limit our discussion of Mr. N's personality to his intelligence. Throughout his life, Mr. N has been an intelligent young man, so he does not appear to rest on the extreme side of this dimension. Also, Mr. N presents with psychiatric symptoms that are not consistent with who he was as a child or adolescent; they are a change from his usual attitude and behavior. As is the case with other individuals who present with bizarre thoughts, feelings, and behavior, the form of Mr. N's illness cannot be explained from the dimensional perspective. Episodic commenting and command hallucinations are not accounted for by the logic of dimensional reasoning, which is based in the recognition of enduring characteristics. Therefore, for the purposes of this discussion, we can conclude that Mr. N's present condition is not arising from who he *is* as a person and so is not best understood by the dimensional perspective.

The Behavior Perspective

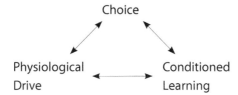

Choice

Physiological Drive ← → Conditioned Learning

If a patient has been engaging in a pattern of repetitive innate or acquired behaviors to achieve a certain end, then his present condition may be explained, in part or wholly, by this perspective. In Mr. N's case, he has engaged and is engaging in a pattern of behaviors, namely daily marijuana use from age 14 to 18, heavy alcohol use for two months at age 18, and twice weekly marijuana use from age 18 to the present. He has used both substances to achieve the desired state of euphoria (i.e., they are goal-oriented behaviors) but also to attempt to escape from the tyranny of the auditory hallucinations. Mr. N's repetitive marijuana smoking is something he's enacting at present to reach a certain end, and may be partially relevant to the origin of his current presentation. Mr. N's psychiatric condition is not explained directly by marijuana dependence, as it is not typical of intoxication or withdrawal related to cannabis use. Nevertheless, certain individuals who use marijuana are at increased risk of developing psychotic illness.[1, 2]

The Disease Perspective

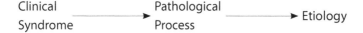

Clinical Syndrome → Pathological Process → Etiology

Based on what we know to date, disease reasoning seems most appropriate to explain Mr. N's illness. In a psychiatric condition best explained by the disease perspective, we assume there is a "broken part," an abnormality in the structure or function of the brain. We can't demonstrate a specific brain abnormality in schizophrenia that is corrected by antipsychotic medication, as we can in the example of diabetes corrected by insulin. However, we observe that Mr. N's auditory hallucinations return after he stopped taking haloperidol. This, coupled with the increasing intensity of the hallucinations over the years in the absence of treatment, suggests a brain disease as an explanation for Mr. N's current presentation. His symptoms have come upon him unbidden, as happens with nonpsychiatric diseases and some psychiatric conditions. Further support for disease reasoning to explain the clinical syndrome of schizophrenia comes from scientific research, including neuroimaging studies, which hint at a distinct pattern of pathologic brain dysfunction and structural disruptions, and animal studies suggesting maldevelopment of the brain as a possible etiology.[3]

Steps 6 and 7: Formulation and Treatment Plan

As with Ms. W in case 1, Mr. N is not a diagnostic dilemma. He presents with the clinical syndrome of schizophrenia, which has been described for centuries and is best understood as something Mr. N *has*. The constellation of signs and symptoms does not appear to be arising from something he has *encountered*, who he *is*, or what he is *doing*. Initially, Mr. N is disorganized in his thought, making the interview a challenge. He offers little spontaneous speech at first and although he later speaks more freely, the content of his speech is vague and without much depth. Mr. N's auditory hallucinations resolve with treatment, but his affect remains flat and he continues to be apathetic, ambivalent, and quietly delusional. He describes a chronic, deteriorating illness characterized primarily by a change in his perceptual experiences and thoughts. On our evaluation he has delusions of grandeur not characteristic of mania. He describes delusions that seem to grow out of an attempt to explain the hallucinatory phenomena he is experiencing. Since we have applied the *Perspectives* approach and can conclude that Mr. N's current condition is best thought of as schizophrenia, a disease for which the pathologic etiology and mechanism are as of yet unknown, resumption of antipsychotic medication is the recommended pharmacologic treatment.

We include Mr. N's case here for several reasons. First, we want to illustrate the axiom that we have found to be most helpful in psychiatric evaluation: "Observations before interpretations." Mr. N's life story records a *sequence* of encounters in a certain *setting:* Mr. N moves to a new country where he has few friends and his mother develops a psychiatric condition requiring hospitalization. Mr. N then develops the onset of auditory hallucinations. It is very tempting, especially for beginners, to link causally a new event to an antecedent event (e.g., onset of hallucinations to relocation and mother's illness). If we interpret Mr. N's current symptoms as arising from his life story, prior to obtaining his and others' historical observations regarding his use of marijuana and the hallucinations' response to haloperidol, and before making our own observations during the history and MSE, we are interpreting before observing. One of the strengths of the *Perspectives* approach is the application of its several concepts in a systematic sequence—thus protecting against the tendency to interpret before observing.

Although Mr. N's auditory hallucinations and delusions are bizarre, and perhaps even the most naïve beginner would not fall prey to using his life story to explain his symptoms, not every case offers this assurance (as we will see in later cases). So, although Mr. N has experienced significant personal life events, the life-story perspective is better used to explain the content and timing of the onset of his illness rather than the illness itself. Whereas the general form of auditory hallucinations (an auditory perception without a stimulus) differs little from patient to patient, the specific form and content of a hallucination can be very personal. The specific form of Mr. N's auditory hallucination, the voice of former Egyptian leader Hosni Mubarak, and its content may be related to Mr. N's past and current life events, such as his Egyptian heritage and the recent revolution in Egypt. This variability in a symptom's specific form and content, shaped by events in a patient's life, is known as the pathoplastic features of the syndrome (versus the more pathognomic aspects of the syndrome, such as the auditory hallucinations themselves). The timing of the onset of Mr. N's hallucinations may also be explained, in part, by life events, such as the stress of the immigration and his mother's illness. Mr. N's continued use of marijuana and his parents' separation, coupled with the lack of insight into his disease, the beneficial effects of antipsychotic treatment, and the consequences of his nonadherence with haloperidol are other life-story factors relevant to his psychiatric conditions.

A second reason for including Mr. N's case is that it demonstrates how behaviors may not only precipitate the onset of disease but may also affect its course. Initiation of marijuana use before age 18 can significantly increase the risk of psychotic symptoms and disorders and decrease the age of onset of schizophrenia.[1, 2] Although we have no way of knowing whether Mr. N's psychiatric symptoms would have had a delayed onset or perhaps would not have developed at all had he never used marijuana or had begun using after the age of 18, there is a clear relationship in population studies between the behavior of marijuana use, especially use prior to the age of 18, and the onset of the disease of schizophrenia.

Case Conclusion

Mr. N agrees to restart his medication. During his hospitalization, he is seen by a nutritionist and his surgeon to address a feeding rehabilitation to facilitate eventual removal of his feeding tube. Subsequently his hallucinations stabilize, and he is discharged home with follow-up with Dr. L and a psychosocial rehabilitation day program. In addition, he commits to abstaining from marijuana use and agrees to submit weekly urine samples to screen for any use.

Summary Points

1 Make observations before interpretations
2 Pathoplastic features arise as personal life-story events shape the pathognomic aspects of a psychiatric syndrome
3 Behaviors can precipitate and sustain psychiatric disease

A Mother's Overdose

Life Story and Dimension

D r. Davis, a psychiatrist at a small academic hospital, receives a call from Darcie, a third-year medical student, asking if he would see her 37-year-old aunt, Melissa E, for a psychiatric evaluation. Darcie described the situation in this way: "My aunt's always been really upbeat and never looked sad or anything. But it turns out she lost her job six months ago and didn't tell anyone. She's been under so much financial stress and it got to the point last week where she took an overdose of zolpidem."

Dr. Davis agrees to see Ms. E and, with her permission, also talks with Ms. E's partner.

(Dr. Davis's comments are printed in *italics*.)

Hello, Ms. E. I'm Dr. Davis. It's a pleasure to meet you.

Thanks for seeing me. You made quite an impression on Darcie. You come highly recommended.

Darcie was wonderful. I really liked working with her. She'll be a great doctor. I'd like to know, however, how you are doing.

I'm fine. I know that when I took those pills, I really scared a lot of people. But, I feel completely back to normal now.

Before we focus on what's been going on recently I'd like first to get to know a bit about who you are as a person and what your life has been like up until now. That way I'll have a context for understanding what happened. Have you ever seen a psychiatrist before?

No, no one thought I needed to until now, I guess.

Did you ever think you needed to see someone?

Never in my wildest dreams. I'm more surprised by what happened than anybody.

Well, again, I'm glad that we will have a chance to talk. Why don't we start with you telling me a little about your parents.

Well, they're getting older but they're still doing fine; I mean, for being in their 70s. They've got a great condo in Charleston.

Do you get to see them often?

Fairly often. They're coming up this weekend to check on me. They're pretty upset about what happened, I guess.

And you mentioned a sister. How is your relationship with her? Do you have any other sisters or brothers?

Nope, it's just the two of us. We're pretty close; she's only 15 months older than me. She's had depression.

Has she seen anyone for that?

Yeah. She was really down in the dumps, especially after her last son was born—she's got four kids—so her obstetrician gave her a medication to help. It's one of the ones that is always on TV. It seemed to do the trick for her.

I see. Any other family history of psychiatric conditions, drug or alcohol problems, suicide attempts . . . ?

Nope. No one except my sister. We never were a family to talk a lot about our feelings.

What about other medical problems in you or in your family?

My mother had to have a pacemaker put in a few years ago, but other than that, no. In general, we're all really healthy.

(Ms. E is asked about and denies any problems during her gestation, infancy, and early childhood.)

Great. What was it like for you growing up?

I was always well behaved. I tried my best to make my parents proud. I went to a private school and got okay grades. I played soccer and was pretty active physically. I didn't drink, smoke, or any of that. My father was ex-military and was pretty strict with us.

Did you date in high school or have a steady partner?

Nah, I mainly hung out with my girlfriends, but that was fine by me. I'm gay, you know.

When were you aware of your sexual orientation?

I think I've known since elementary school. I remember having crushes on my first and third grade teachers—both women. And then in high school when the other girls were mooning over Johnny Depp, I was dreaming of Madonna. I think everyone knew, really. Even my father didn't seem surprised when I told them.

When was that?

My senior year. They were riding me about getting a date for the prom. I just couldn't take it any longer and told them.

What did you do after high school?

I went straight to Virginia Tech and got a business degree. I really loved it there. After I graduated, I stayed on working in their accounting department—until two years ago when I got my job with the video game company.

I know you said in high school you stayed away from alcohol, smoking, etc. What about in college?

There was one semester, fall of junior year, when I drank quite a bit. It got to a point where I was drinking a couple of beers a day. I realized I was starting to gain some weight, so I just stopped.

Did you have a problem stopping? Or get into any trouble due to your drinking?

No, I never got into any trouble. I was usually just hanging out with friends after dinner. I never even went to the big parties. As soon as I realized I was gaining weight I stopped, never noticed any problems.

Did you ever notice your hands shaking or a craving for alcohol?

No, nothing like that.

And drugs?

I never used any drugs—I don't believe in them. And I haven't even had much to drink since college. I like to run and keep my head clear.

That's good to hear. Can you tell me about your partner? Where'd you meet?

Sure. I met Sherry at Virginia Tech our junior year and we moved in together right after graduating. She's the only person I've ever been with, you know. We've been very happy together until now. She's still pretty angry about what happened, which I don't really understand. We didn't lose our house or anything. I guess she's upset I didn't tell her about losing my job. I'm upset about that, too.

Do you have any children?

One girl and two boys: our daughter, Cassie, is 11, and our sons, Robbie and Ken, are 9 and 7. Sherry's brother is the father, the sperm donor. Our kids are doing great—they're very well behaved and get good grades in school. Sherry stayed at home with them when they were little, but she went back to work—teaching—after we moved here and our youngest started pre-K.

Did she like being at home?

She was glad to get a little break from the classroom, for sure, but, after three kids, I think she was ready to go back.

She likes her work?

You know, she really does. She loves working with middle schoolers and her principal is terrific. It's a terrific school.

And you were working for a video game company?

I was. It was a really amazing company. So amazing that they got bought up by the biggest game company in the country. That company already had a full accounting staff, so I got the ax. I really loved that job, plus it was the whole reason we moved here and bought this house. I was making more money than I ever thought I would and I liked being in the entertainment business a lot. It was a big change from Virginia Tech.

That's right. You were at Virginia Tech during the shootings, then? That must have been a frightening experience.

I was in the building next door and could hear the gunfire. It was traumatic: hearing the screams, seeing the helicopters, being on lockdown, looking out my window and watching the bodies being carried out. There was lots of crying. And, the looks on everyone's faces . . .

You were really pretty close then. What do you mean by traumatic?

I don't know, really; that's what everybody said.

Well, how did it affect you? Did you have trouble sleeping? Nightmares?

No, but I've always been able to handle things pretty well, so it didn't seem strange to me that I didn't seem too bothered by it. I know everybody thinks it's kind of weird that I never talked about it. But, what was there to say? It's a terrible tragedy, for sure, but . . . the guy killed himself so it's not like it's going to happen again. I think Sherry was more upset than I was, and she wasn't even there. I felt sorry for the kids and their families and all. But, I mean, it wasn't like I was in the same building or anything.

But you were really close to the shootings.

Yeah, I was. They eventually evacuated my building, the whole campus. I went home and watched the rest of it on TV. It was a pretty extreme thing—I recognize that. That guy must have been crazy. I was just glad more people weren't hurt. And, I felt sorry for the parents of the kids. But I didn't cry or anything. And I never felt afraid for myself.

(Ms. E is asked about and denies any medical conditions, surgeries, medications, and drug allergies.)

I've got a few more specific questions for you that will help me understand you better.

Sure.

Would you say you're a generally optimistic or pessimistic person?

That's easy—my family always calls me the eternal optimist and they are so right.

Do you tend to be suspicious or are you a trusting person?

Oh, definitely trusting. I always think everyone has my best interest in mind. . . . I guess it's from growing up in the South where everyone's so friendly and good hearted.

Do you consider yourself a moody person, or are you more even-tempered?

Even-tempered for sure. I'm very laid back and easy-going.

Are you much of a worrier or more carefree?

Well, Sherry sure thinks I should have worried a little more. No, like I say, I never let much get to me.

Are you able to express your feelings fairly easily or are you more controlled?

I think I'm pretty much in the middle there.

Do you think of yourself as more dependent or independent?

I'm not sure; I guess pretty independent. I like to pull myself up by my own boot straps. I'm not a complainer.

Are you cautious or impulsive?

I think I'm in the middle there too.

Are you generous or frugal?

Definitely generous. I think that's part of my problem . . .

Do you think of yourself as more of a leader or a follower?

Maybe a little bit more of a leader.

Are you a solitary type of person or more sociable?

I'm pretty social. I don't get wild or anything, but I like being around people. I like going to parties, entertaining, and what not.

Do you consider yourself a patient person or impatient?

With three kids, you have to be patient. I stay pretty calm despite what they're getting into. Sherry and I are both really patient people, I think.

Are you strict or easy-going?

With the kids?

Yes, and in general?

Well, I guess we spoil them some—with toys and games and all that. But we always have dinner together every night and are pretty strict when it comes to letting them watch TV, setting regular bed-times, those sorts of things. They know not to talk back to us, although we don't believe in corporal punishment. I think we're stricter with our kids than most of our friends are. But I don't think we're overly strict and all, in general. Like I said, I'm pretty laid back.

Are you a confident person or do you doubt yourself?

I'm usually pretty confident.

Are you dependable and reliable or more unreliable?

I'm definitely reliable.

Are you an anxious person or calm?

My friends always say I'm so calm with my kids. No, I don't worry much at all. I'm definitely calm. My sister thinks I should worry more!

Are you a pretty sensitive person or do you have a thick skin?

I'm probably somewhere in the middle there; maybe a little on the thick-skin side, I guess.

Are you neat or messy?

Oh, you have to be pretty organized to be an accountant. At least I am. But, I'm not a neat freak or anything. I just like things to be where I can find them.

Are you a self-conscious person or do you not care that much about what other people think?

Hmmm. I think I'm somewhere in the middle there. Well, no, I don't think I'm very self-conscious, no.

I appreciate your answering all of my questions. I am going to ask you one last, broad question. Can you tell me about what's been happening more recently? Tell me as much as you are willing to right now. We can always revisit it later.

Well . . . the easiest way to start is to say that I'm used to handling my own problems. I tried to handle this problem on my own and failed. When the game company was bought out, they let me go, and I decided not to tell Sherry. It's as simple as that.

When were you laid off?

Six months ago. I was sure I was going to be able to get another job and was planning to tell her as soon as I got another job.

She thought you were still going to work?

I know. But it wasn't that bad. It wasn't like I pretended to leave the house or anything. And work was casual so I didn't have to dress up in the morning. She left the house before I did and we never talked much about my work anyway. The kids keep us pretty busy.

But you weren't getting a paycheck?

No, but being an accountant, I have always managed the finances for the family, so Sherry knew to let me handle it unless I asked for help, which I never did. We'd moved, bought a new house, probably more house than we needed. The house was in my name, but Sherry gave me some money each month for the payment, plus we had our student loans, credit card debt. . . . I tried to juggle everything for a while, but I knew it was only a matter of time before we wouldn't be able to make our house payment. And eventually the creditors started calling. Then, last week, the bank threatened to take the house—they are being very tough nowadays.

Did you ever discuss this with Sherry?

No. I didn't want her to worry and I was sure I was going to find a job and fix it all somehow. It's not like I was gambling, doing anything illegal, or blowing money. I just kept thinking, "Somehow, I'll figure it out . . . I always do." But when the bank called, I realized I couldn't fix things and I was going to have to tell Sherry everything.

She really didn't know anything?

Not a bit. I was sure I was going to be able to get a job and figure everything out. I know it sounds crazy, but that's what I thought. But when the bank called, I started to panic. I didn't sleep well that night and I couldn't figure a way out. The next morning, I just wanted to make it all go away, and so I took some of Sherry's sleeping pills.

Zolpidem?

Right.

How many did you take?

However many were left in the bottle. I'm not sure. Maybe twenty . . . I don't know. Sherry uses them sometimes when she has trouble getting to sleep, which isn't very often.

Were you trying to kill yourself?

I don't think so. I didn't want to die. I mean I love her and the kids too much to do that. That's why I took the pills. I was so ashamed. I just couldn't deal with telling them.

So, what happened after you took the pills?

I went to the bed and fell asleep. The next thing I remember is being in the emergency room. Sherry had come home with the kids and found me passed out. She's the one who called the ambulance. They took me to the hospital, and I was in the psych ward for two days.

How are your children doing?

They're worried about me. I really regret them seeing all that. That's what I feel most bad about now. The good news is the truth is out, and I'm happy about that.

You said you didn't sleep well that night. Had you been having trouble with your sleep or appetite in the months leading up to this?

No, I've always been a really good sleeper. Except for that one night when I didn't sleep so well. I've always been able to eat.

What about your energy level, had that changed?

No, I went running the morning before and felt as good as always. Really, nothing was bothering me until the bank called.

What about your concentration?

That's been fine.

And had you been feeling worse about yourself before the over-dose? Not that you should, but did you feel like a bad person or a failure in any way?

No. Like I said, I thought it would all work out and that a new job was right around the corner. But it's a tough time to get work. And, once the bank called, I realized I couldn't keep up the charade any longer. I felt bad. Like I'd failed my kids, my family. That's why I did what I did. I just couldn't face letting them down.

You said you panicked that morning, but had you been feeling at all worried or anxious before then?

No. Not a bit. No one seems to believe me when I say I really thought it would all work out, but it's true.

I know you hadn't told your partner about this because you didn't want her to worry, but had you confided in anyone?

No. Sherry's my best friend. I never tell anyone something that I wouldn't tell her.

(With Ms. E's permission, Dr. Davis speaks with her partner, Ms. G, on the telephone while Ms. E is excused to the waiting room. Ms. G confirms that her partner is an optimistic, trusting, easy-going, independent, generous, confident, calm, and organized individual. Ms. G says that, although the patient is carefree, she is not typically reckless or impulsive. Ms. G thinks of Ms. E as a "stoic" person who copes "almost too well" with events, including the incident at Virginia Tech. Ms. G confirms that her partner is not misusing or abusing any illicit or licit substances.)

Ms. G, I was wondering if you could give me your perspective on what's been happening.

Until last week, I thought everything was fine. Things were hectic, with the kids and work, but nothing seemed out of the ordinary at all. She seemed the same as always. Nothing unusual.

Had you noticed any change in her sleep or eating at all?

No. She always sleeps like a rock—better than I do. And she's a great cook and makes wonderful meals for us, which she always eats, too. I think that's why she runs, so she can eat anything she wants to. And she does.

And so what happened that morning? What was she like?

Well, she seemed a little quiet, and I asked if she was feeling okay. I thought she might have been feeling sick or something. But she said she was fine, and that was that. I kissed her goodbye, like usual, and then the kids and I left to go to school.

And then?

I came home and she was passed out on the bed. The empty medicine bottle was there and I called an ambulance and, at the hospital, they decided she needed to be admitted to the psych unit. And that's when she told me what had happened—that she'd lost her job.

And?

And I was furious. I still am furious. I can't believe it! Luckily, my parents helped us out so we could keep the house, but . . . I can't believe she lied to me about going to work and didn't look upset or anything. I really don't understand how she could keep that from me. What was she thinking?

You sound pretty angry.

Damn straight. I'm seeing someone now just to deal with this. I don't know if I can forgive her for this. I just don't understand . . .

MSE: Ms. E is a well-groomed, alert, and cooperative woman who appears her stated age. She sits quietly in her chair and makes good eye contact throughout the interview with no tremors or tics. Her gait is assessed as normal. There are no apparent hallucinations. She answers all questions appropriately, without delay, mostly giving to-the-point answers. She makes little small talk and speaks with a fairly monotonous tone, with her speech normal in amount and volume. There is no evidence of thought disorder or aphasia. She describes her mood as "fine" and her affect is neutral and constricted. She denies any suicidal or homicidal thoughts. She feels some guilt about her suicide attempt and her debt but is not delusional about these matters. She is not hopeless and denies grandiose or persecutory delusions. There are no hallucinations, obsessions, compulsions, or phobias. She is fully oriented and has a good fund of knowledge with an MMSE score of 30/30. Her intelligence is assessed as above average. Her insight is poor into the potential impact of her deception on her relationship with her partner, and her judgment is poor regarding her decision to take an overdose of pills rather than talk to her partner and ask for her help.

The Discussion

Steps 2–4: History, MSE, and Collateral Information

Ms. E is the younger of two children, born into a stable and relatively affluent family. Her childhood and adolescence were not marked by any extreme events or chronic family discord. She was a good student, played on the soccer team, dated a few boys in high school but was not sexually active, and avoided alcohol and drugs. She was neither particularly impulsive nor overly cautious. She was apparently able to negotiate the normal developmental challenges of adolescence, as well as her awareness of her homosexual orientation, with emotional stability. At college, she engaged briefly in some binge-drinking behavior, but stopped drinking when she realized she was gaining weight. She did well in her business courses at college, and was sociable, meeting her partner during their junior year. Since graduating from college, Ms. E has been steadily employed as an accountant and now has three children ranging in age from 7 to 11 years. Over the past fifteen years, she has weathered all of her life transitions (e.g., adulthood, domestic partnership, motherhood, employment) with her characteristic stoicism and optimism. Her niece and partner both note their surprise at her reaction to the massacre that happened at her place of work, a mass-shooting in which thirty-two people were killed and many others wounded.

Two years after that event, Ms. E changed jobs and moved to a new state with her family, where she bought a home. Despite losing her job and confronting growing financial debt, Ms. E suffered no change in her appetite, libido, mood, energy/motivation, concentration, or view of herself or her future. She continued to enjoy a near-daily run, including one she took on the day before her overdose. She had no problems sleeping until the night before, when she described the onset of worry after the bank called and threatened foreclosure on their home. She had no thoughts of harming herself, however, until the next morning when she took an overdose of zolpidem with the hopes of escaping telling her partner and children about her job loss six months prior and the resultant financial problems.

Step 5: Consideration from Each Perspective

The Life-Story Perspective

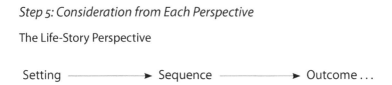

Until the massacre at Virginia Tech, Ms. E had never encountered any out-of-the-ordinary stressor. However, on the day of the shootings, she directly and personally witnessed the sequelae of an event that resulted in the death and injury of many people (and could have resulted in her own death or injury). The extreme nature of the event and her close proximity to it qualifies as a trauma experience according to the *DSM-IV-TR*, and Ms. E is able to voice an understanding of the theoretically traumatic nature of the event. However, Ms. E's response did not involve intense fear, helplessness, or horror, and so does not meet *DSM-IV-TR* criteria for a traumatic exposure; nor does Ms. E describe distressing memories, dreams, or flashbacks of the event.

More recently, Ms. E lost her job and experienced growing financial difficulties, resulting in the potential loss of the home she shares with her female partner and three children. Although this stressor is more ordinary than the massacre at Virginia Tech and is not of a life-threatening nature, it is one that would cause most people to feel worried, helpless, and embarrassed. In addition, it is a stressor in which Ms. E is personally involved and for which she is partly responsible. However, Ms. E did not feel any of these emotions until the bank called the day before the overdose. Despite the absence of emotional distress until less than a day prior to her overdose, Ms. E's overdose did occur in the *setting* of job loss and financial problems that she had hidden from her partner. Although she had encountered a major potentially traumatic event in the past without emotional distress and has endured six months of job loss and growing financial problems, her overdose seems related to the bank's threat of foreclosure. If these symptoms are arising from what she's *encountered* in her life, they would be best treated with the construction of a plausible, chronological, coherent narrative. Although her current psychiatric condition may be the result of what she has *encountered*, her overdose does not seem to fit with how she reacted to stresses in the past, nor has impulsivity been a problematic behavior through the months she has been without a job and facing financial difficulties, and so we will defer a conclusion regarding the contribution of her life story to her psychiatric condition until we've fully considered her problem from the other three perspectives.

The Dimensional Perspective

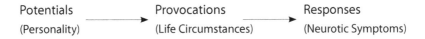

Potentials → Provocations → Responses
(Personality)   (Life Circumstances)   (Neurotic Symptoms)

Ms. E does not appear to rest at an extreme on any cognitive dimension and her intelligence is unlikely to be playing a role in the origin of her present distress. But what about the psychological dimension of temperament? Do aspects of Ms. E's temperament have anything to do with her presentation?

Just as the cognitive dimension of intelligence can be measured and recorded for an individual as a point on the WAIS Full-Scale IQ, so can a temperament dimension, such as introversion or extraversion, be measured and recorded for an individual. And, just as with the Full-Scale IQ, where an individual rests on the introversion-extraversion dimension is relatively stable over time, presuming no supervening process like dementia or major depression.[1] A thorough history and MSE can yield enough information to allow a clinician to estimate an individual's intelligence and temperament. In the case of Ms. E, based on her school performance, occupational attainment, and vocabulary, we have estimated her intelligence to be above average. We can also approximate her temperament based on her and her family's reports of her (which have not been included in their entirety here for brevity's sake) before the present illness. This baseline temperament is also known as her "premorbid personality," making the point that "morbid" psychiatric conditions can have an impact on the appearance of an individual's personality. (A person in the throes of nicotine withdrawal may appear uncharacteristically short-tempered, for example.)

Although a formal measurement of temperament is not always feasible and/or necessary in the clinical setting, the Neuroticism, Extraversion, Openness Personality Inventory (NEO-PI)[1] is a test that we have found to be clinically useful at times. The NEO-PI can reliably and validly measure five aspects of temperament. Full presentation of the NEO-PI is beyond the scope of this discussion. Of relevance is that the five dimensions of temperament that the NEO-PI measures are neuroticism, extraversion, openness, agreeableness, and conscientiousness. For the purpose of introducing the concept of temperament to the beginner and to simplify the discussion, in this case book we focus on two of these dimensions: introversion-extraversion and neuroticism-stability.

Introversion-extraversion and neuroticism-stability as dimensions of temperament were described by Wilhelm Wundt and Carl Jung, verified by Hans Eysenck in a male military population,[2] and replicated by Costa[1] and others. We will consider each of these dimensional axes separately, beginning with introversion-extraversion. This dimension separates individuals on the basis of their *potential* vulnerability to *respond* maladaptively to certain *provocations*. Introverts tend to consider the past or future implications of an event and to have a slower emotional reaction to events.[3] Extraverts' emotional responses are the opposite. They tend to focus more on the present than past or future and to have quick emotional reactions to events. An introverted individual is more apt to consider the consequences of things done or said in the past, and/or things to be said or done in the future (e.g., a remark made at a party, an upcoming exam, the road not taken) and is slow to warm up to others. An extraverted individual is less prone to worry about the consequences of what she's said/done or is going to say/do and is, thus, more apt to be comfortable in social situations and view herself as "happy-go-lucky." Emotional *responses* come fast for extraverts but usually are forgotten as quickly as they come.

Introverts aren't inherently "better" than extraverts (or vice versa), but each can be *potentially* vulnerable in the setting of specific *provocations*. For instance, an introvert may not be the life of the party because she is reflecting on the consequences of a conversation or action, and so is less spontaneous socially. However, this reflection may help an introvert avoid certain impulsive actions, thus avoiding some troubles. Besides being fun at parties, an extravert may be well suited to certain careers, like sales. Most extraverts, in the face of forty-nine "cold calls" resulting in no sales, can still make that fiftieth call. Being present-oriented, however, an extravert can make impulsive decisions that get her into trouble.

Ms. E's temperament does not appear to be on either extreme of the introversion-extraversion dimension. Her history contains evidence that she was able to set long-term goals relating to academics, athletics, and training and did not allow life events to distract her from these goals. She successfully avoided making unhealthy decisions regarding alcohol and drug use in high school and was never promiscuous. However, she has enough present-orientation to have enjoyed being part of a social group in college, where she drank alcohol to intoxication and met her future partner. Her niece describes her as a cheerful, upbeat individual, an opinion with which Ms. E's partner concurs.

The midpoint of this dimension is stability, with neuroticism (instability) and great stability lying on either extreme. The term *neurotic* has been over-used in popular culture, loaded with other connotations, and rendered relatively meaningless. We prefer to use the word neurotic to describe an individual prone to experiencing strong negative affect. This dimension has also been referred to as the unstable-stable and strong-weak dimension of temperament.[3] We have found that it is most easily grasped by students when described as the instability–great stability dimension.

This dimension distinguishes individuals on the strength of their emotional responses to life events. We consider *instability* to mean the tendency to respond very strongly and *great stability* to mean the tendency to respond very weakly, and so will use this definition to describe this dimension.[3] As Ms. E's case illustrates so well, however, placement on either of these dimensional extremes can render one vulnerable to responding problematically to certain provocations (although being on the great stability side is less likely to provoke a problematic response and much less likely to prompt a psychiatric referral).

Ms. E does not appear to rest on either extreme of the introversion-extraversion dimension. She seems to be more extraverted than introverted, but not extremely so. She is described as warm and views herself as sociable, but has demonstrated, in a variety of settings, her ability to steer a steady future-oriented course in life, without being swept up by present circumstances. She is not quick to anger, nor is she slow or cool in her emotional response to others.

Although Ms. E does not appear to lie on either extreme of the introversion-extraversion dimension, the same cannot be said for her position on the instability–great stability dimension. The strength of Ms. E's emotional responses to both normal and extraordinary life events, such as the campus shootings, tends to be relatively weak. Her family was perplexed because they viewed the shootings as a severely stressful event for which she should have had a stronger reaction. However, one study suggests that those shootings did not produce strong emotional responses in everyone, and that individuals responded to that event in a variety of ways.[4] Ms. E's niece and partner describe her as upbeat, stoic, and optimistic. She describes herself as optimistic, laid back, and easy-going. Her history suggests that Ms. E is an individual who tends to have less intense emotions than others, which has served her well in many circumstances, including the campus shootings.

How does an understanding of Ms. E's temperament as somewhat extraverted and greatly stable help us understand the secrecy in which she kept her job loss and growing financial problems and her overdose when the secret was threatened with exposure? Neither she nor her family describes a life-long pattern of secrecy, excessive independence, or overestimation of her own abilities. Her secrecy appears to have arisen, rather, from her general sense of optimism and low level of worry. A tendency toward emotionally weak responses to life events does not usually compel someone to seek help. Had Ms. E's partner discovered sooner that she was keeping her job loss and subsequent financial difficulties from her, she may have sought psychiatric treatment for them as a couple. However, she did not become aware of her secrecy until Ms. E had taken the overdose of pills.

The Behavior Perspective

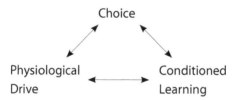

In Ms. E's case, she denies any use of illicit substances and now only rarely drinks alcohol. She has no evidence of primary sleep or sexual disorders. Some recurrent suicide attempts are learned repetitive behaviors that have qualities of an acquired drive. Although Ms. E's overdose is an isolated behavior, it is an act with the apparent goal of avoiding telling her partner the truth about her job loss and financial difficulties. This perspective does not account for the origin of the distress that precipitated the overdose. An overdose is a behavior, however, and therefore the behavior perspective is applicable to this aspect of the case. Why Ms. E did what she did (as opposed to doing something else, like asking for help)—the choice she made—is relevant to the formulation of her case, even though the origin of her presentation cannot be fully explained by the behavioral perspective.

The Disease Perspective

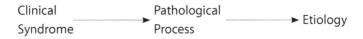

Ms. E has had no syndromic change in her thoughts, mood, or behavior. We do not see her current psychiatric condition as representing a new theme in her life and are unable to understand it as arising from an abnormality in the structure or function of her brain (something that she *has*). Because Ms. E is not exhibiting any clinical psychiatric syndrome such as a mood disorder or schizophrenia, the disease perspective does not explain the origin of her current problems.

Steps 6 and 7: Formulation and Treatment Plan

By taking a thorough history, we are able to put Ms. E's presentation in the context of the history of psychiatric diseases her family *has,* what Ms. E herself has *encountered* in her life, what she *does,* and who she intellectually and emotionally *is* in the world. Ms. E's psychiatric symptoms, signs, and course fulfill *DSM* criteria for an adjustment disorder. The circumstances of her life that led up to the acute distress and overdose are relevant to her present illness. We can construct a meaningful narrative to explain her distress and overdose as arising from her life circumstances. The *setting* of the narrative is based on an understanding of her as a person (i.e., the dimensional perspective). The *sequence* of the narrative would begin with her growing financial pressures and her failed attempt to deal with them in secret, and the *outcome* would be the overdose as seen from her point of view.

Although she does not meet *DSM* criteria for a personality disorder, aspects of her personality do come into play in this presentation. She was able to shrug off exposure to a severely stressful event and finesse her more recent job loss and financial problems—until she was not able to.

When foreclosure was threatened, she chose to avoid telling her partner the truth by taking an overdose. Applying the *Perspectives* approach allows us to see that Ms. E has an extremely stable temperament. This adaptive psychological quality, however, leads Ms. E to be *vulnerable* to a lack of emotional *response* to certain life events, events that would typically *provoke* a response in most individuals, leading them to seek help.

After considering Ms. E's presentation from all four perspectives, we conclude that the dimensional and life-story perspectives offer the most coherent ways to understand her. Individual psychotherapy with the goal of guiding a patient through life events is the indicated treatment for patients with dimensional conditions. Although Dr. Davis knows that psychotherapy that generates little emotional arousal is unlikely to succeed,[5] he hopes that, with an experienced and skillful psychotherapist to guide her, Ms. E may achieve some success. Dr. Davis recommends weekly individual psychotherapy sessions for Ms. E to focus on helping Ms. E understand why her partner is so upset with her secrecy and overdose, and to generate longer-term goals, such as to be less secretive and more likely to seek help in the future. To that end, the psychiatrist persuades Ms. E to have periodic discussions with her partner about their life together, even though Ms. E doesn't feel anything is wrong. In addition, Dr. Davis refers both Ms. E and her partner to couples psychotherapy to help address the issues surrounding the broken trust.

Case Conclusion

Ms. E enters treatment remorseful regarding her secrecy about the job loss, the financial problems, and the effect her overdose had on the immediate family. Once others become aware of the problem, they offer financial help. With the crisis of foreclosure averted, Ms. E's distress vanishes. She is sleeping and eating well, has a good mood, feels confident, and is optimistic about the future. She has trouble appreciating why her partner remains angry and distrustful toward her. The initial focus of the psychotherapy is to help Ms. E understand why her partner is so upset with her secrecy and overdose and to generate longer-term goals, such as to be less secretive with her partner. However, Ms. E feels little need for ongoing psychiatric treatment.

Although attempts are made to engage her in individual psychotherapy, her level of emotional arousal is so low that it becomes apparent that individual psychotherapy is of little benefit. From Ms. E's point of view, her problems are now behind her and so is her distress. Ms. E is ready to return to looking for a job and the rest of her life as if nothing happened. She is referred to couples therapy in hopes of gaining a better understanding of the impact of her actions (or lack thereof) on her partner and their relationship, but she is not interested in couples therapy and her partner does not insist that they go to treatment together. With Ms. E's consent, Dr. Davis talks with her family to help them better understand Ms. E's temperament so that they can appreciate its strengths as well as its vulnerabilities. With this education, they can accept her lack of emotional response to certain situations and recognize situations for which they may need to be more vigilant. This way they can adapt to her temperament, rather than expecting her to react in a particular way to an event. Ms. E stopped coming to individual psychotherapy after less than a half-dozen sessions, because she was no longer feeling distressed.

Summary Points

1 Introversion-extraversion and instability–great stability are two dimensions that measure fundamental aspects of temperament

2 Resting on the extreme end of a dimension, even great stability, can render one vulnerable to responding problematically to certain provocations

3 Some degree of emotional arousal is necessary for successful psychotherapy

A Man with Depression amidst Multiple Life Stressors

Life Story or Disease?

D r. Cohen, a consultation-liaison psychiatrist, is asked to see Mr. Samuel R, a 48-year-old counselor, after a nurse found the patient weeping in his hospital room following right knee replacement surgery.

(Dr. Cohen's comments are in *italics*.)

Dr. J asked me to see you because he was concerned about your mood. How have you been doing?

I've been having a rough time. There's been so much going on. . . . I'm not sure exactly where I should start.

Let's start with your family history. Are your parents still living?

My mother died when I was 7. She had a heart attack.

I'm sorry to hear that. How about your father?

He's still living, but we haven't talked for years.

I'm sorry. What was it like for you as a child, then, after your mother died?

My father remarried three years after she died, and so my brother and I lived with them. Then my stepmother had the girls.

Tell me a little more about your siblings.

My brother and I are really close. He's only a year older. He's in California now, but we still talk all the time. I don't really know my half-sisters that well.

Has anyone in your family ever seen a psychiatrist?

Nobody in my immediate family ever needed to—not even my

brother after his girlfriend died. But two of my mother's cousins have been depressed—one's on lithium and the other takes an antidepressant, but I'm not sure what it is.

(The patient is asked about and denies any problems during gestation, infancy, and early childhood except for asthma, beginning at age 6, for which hospitalization was not required.)

You mentioned your father remarried and had other children. What was it like growing up with a blended family?

The worst part of growing up, besides my mother dying, was my stepmother—the wicked witch. I was 10 when she came to live with us. I always thought we were good kids, but she hated me and my brother. She just didn't like boys, I think. When I was 15, my dad sent us away to live with our mother's brother. It was crowded there with their three kids, but it was heaven compared to living with her. My aunt and uncle welcomed us with open arms. Their kids were like little brothers and sisters to me. I never saw my dad much after he sent us away.

What did you do after high school?

Well, my dad never gave us a penny for college, so I put myself through school and eleven years later finally got a BA in psychology. I'm working on my master's in social work now. After my BA, I worked as a therapist at the children's hospital in Philadelphia, but since I've been here, I've been working in the Peds department.

And are you in a relationship now?

I was engaged once—to a grad student in philosophy. She was brilliant. We were together for about sixteen years. I put her through grad school and then law school. Then, a couple of years after finishing, she dumped me. I can't say I've been interested in anyone since. It crushed me. I haven't even wanted sex since then.

Do you drink or smoke?

I almost never drink. I've never smoked or used drugs. My biggest vice is my three cups of coffee a day.

Any other medical problems, besides asthma?

All my medical problems are because of this weight; I'm only 5′11″ but I'm over 300 pounds now. That's why I got arthritis in my knees and needed this surgery—from carrying around all this extra weight.

I'm also taking two medications for high blood pressure, insulin for diabetes, my cholesterol is high, and I can't walk without getting out of breath.

I'm sorry to hear all that.

I've just got to lose weight. I tried group therapy, but it didn't help.

I want to shift gears a bit now and ask you a little about what you're like as a person and what your interests are. Are you usually a cheerful/optimistic person or more somber/pessimistic?

How I am now, doc—this isn't me. I'm usually real upbeat. I get along with everybody. I'm usually a rock. I can be a little shy and self-conscious, especially around women. I've been called "sensitive," for better or worse. And I've always been a bit of a perfectionist. I like reading and listening to music. They relax me. I was raised Catholic and try to go to mass as often as I can. I've taught catechism class at church for years.

I understand that you've never seen a psychiatrist before, but I'm wondering if you ever felt like you needed to.

Well, I probably should have seen someone when I was in college. That was when my cousin died. He was only 19 when he fell asleep at the wheel. It was the same year our grandmother died. I was really in a funk then. I couldn't do my work. I even considered dropping out of school.

Did you talk to anyone at all? Did you see a counselor yourself?

No. I should have, I know. It's like the shoemaker's children. But I just got over it and was fine, until my fiancée broke it off.

And so how have things been for you more recently? You moved to Buffalo after that relationship ended?

Yep. It took a while, but I started feeling better—a new job, a new apartment, new friends, new life. I was feeling that my life was getting back on track. I still felt down about my weight, but other than that—and my arthritis and all—life was good. Then two years ago, my uncle that raised me had a stroke. And then, around the same time, my 13-year-old niece was diagnosed with colon cancer. And, if that wasn't enough, my cousin, who's a nurse—the one with bipolar disorder—was accused of harming a patient. I just lost it. I remember being locked out of my apartment—twice I lost my keys—and just not being able to cope. I just sat at the door in a daze. I wasn't think-ing clearly. I was feeling tired all the time, unmotivated. I even dropped out of my master's program.

This all sounds so distressing. How did you deal with those losses?

I guess not too well. I tried going to my GP and he prescribed a sleeping medication—but I hated it. It made me feel awful. I never took another one of those. When I went back, he started me on par-oxetine 20 mg. That was about ten months ago. I didn't put a whole lot of stock in the medication. I really think I should be able to handle things. I mean, I'm a therapist; I should be able to figure things out. And I kept going to work, but all I'd do when I'd come home was eat and go to bed. I don't do anything around the house any more. My apartment is disgusting. The master bedroom sheets got so filthy, I couldn't sleep in the bed. I'm embarrassed to say this but, instead of changing the sheets, I just moved to the other bedroom.

How has your sleep been?

I don't have any trouble falling asleep—I just konk out on the couch every night. But I wake up way too early in the morning and can't get back to sleep. I thought a sleeping pill would help, but it didn't. I'm also eating a lot of junk food, which is a really bad idea.

And your mood?

I'm a little crabby, but mostly I just feel blah. I'm ashamed to say I cry myself to sleep at night. I used to read before bed, but I don't want to read anymore, and I'm not sure if I could. I don't have the energy to do anything. I even stopped teaching Sunday school.

(With Mr. R's permission, Dr. Cohen talks, via telephone, to Mr. R's brother in California who confirms many details of the history, including that his brother is usually a fairly happy-go-lucky but conscientious person.)

MSE: Mr. R is a well-groomed, obese, alert, and cooperative man who appears slightly younger than his age. He makes good eye contact and demonstrates no tics or tremor. There is no evidence of hallucinations. He speaks a moderate amount and responds to questions without delay. His speech is normal in rate, amount, and volume. It is not circumstantial and there is no evidence of thought disorder or apha-sia. He describes his mood as "a little depressed," and he appears sad. His affect is moderately constricted but appropriate to speech content. He denies any suicidal or homicidal thoughts. He has some feelings of guilt and self-blame, especially as related to his eating and body image. He is not hopeless and has no grandiose or persecutory delusions. He has no hallucinations, obsessions, compulsions, or phobias. He is fully oriented and has a good fund of information, with an MMSE score of 30/30. His intelligence is assessed to be above average, and his insight and judgment are normal.

The Discussion

Steps 2–4: History, MSE, and Collateral Informants

Since losing his mother at the age of 7, Mr. R has faced many challenges. Until recently he weathered these difficulties by staying focused on his goals. Mr. R has never used any illicit substance and does not regularly drink alcohol. Although his lifelong struggle with obesity has affected his health, he has not become preoccupied with his weight to the neglect of personal, social, or professional activities. (This is a good example of an aspect of the presentation that may be relevant to our understanding of Mr. R as an individual but does not have a strong bearing, if any, on his current presentation. As such, this is not an issue that we would insist on addressing in individual psychotherapy, except at the patient's request.) Mr. R has had loss of libido since his fiancée left. In the *setting* of multiple personal losses, he describes the gradual emergence of new symptoms over the past two years. Despite his best efforts to persevere in the face of several unexpected tragedies, he has experienced an insidious, yet dramatic, decline in his vital sense (exhibiting poor sleep, appetite, energy/ motivation, and concentration) as well as the symptoms of low mood and decreased self-attitude. These changes were preceded by illnesses in two members of his close extended family and continued in the presence of new and ongoing stressors. After almost a year of 20 mg paroxetine daily, his symptoms have not improved.

Step 5: Consideration from Each Perspective

The Life-Story Perspective

Setting ⎯⎯⎯⎯⎯⎯→ Sequence ⎯⎯⎯⎯⎯⎯→ Outcome ...

This perspective holds great appeal to us humans. Every culture tells stories. We all grow up telling stories. Stories are how we account for what we do. Constructing a meaningful narrative to explain life events, and the behaviors and feelings these events provoke, helps us make sense of our lives and has adaptive value. By bringing a sense of order and control to our external and internal worlds, we are better able to cope with stressors and adapt. Like all of us, Mr. R had used these meaningful explanations repeatedly and successfully throughout his life. In this case, we must strongly consider the life-story perspective as a way of understanding Mr. R's present symptoms. Although he has endured a number of severe childhood stressors, both psychological and physical, his symptoms have followed on the heels of more recent challenges in his life—illnesses and severe legal problems of loved ones. He has had the resilience and optimism to overcome countless adversities in the past, and his current symptoms could be related to these more recent stressors and/or past adversities. If these symptoms are arising from what he's *encountered* in his life, they would be best treated with the construction of a plausible, chronological, coherent narrative. Although his current psychiatric condition may be the result of what he has *encountered*, his current mood does not fit with how he reacted to stresses in the past, and so we will defer a conclusion regarding the origin of his psychiatric condition until we've fully considered his problem from the other perspectives.

The Dimensional Perspective

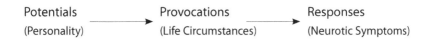

Potentials ⎯⎯⎯⎯⎯→ Provocations ⎯⎯⎯⎯⎯→ Responses
(Personality)   (Life Circumstances)   (Neurotic Symptoms)

Mr. R appears to be of above-average intelligence, although not in the gifted range. His temperament appears to be on neither extreme of the introversion-extraversion dimension. He describes himself at baseline as a cheerful and optimistic individual who is neither totally carefree nor a worrier. He may be more on the instability side of the instability–great stability dimension, as he says that he's a sensitive person but that his moods are relatively stable. Mr. R's ability to navigate all the obstacles that life threw his way is most likely due to his innate intellectual and mood characteristics. Mr. R is an intelligent, easy-going, conscientious individual who seems to be well aware of his strengths and has leveraged them in weathering adversities. Because Mr. R did not describe or demonstrate any tendency toward the extreme in either cognition or temperament (confirmed by an outside informant) and because he successfully weathered so many challenges in the past, we conclude that Mr. R's present condition is not arising from who he *is* as a person, and so cannot be understood primarily by the dimensional perspective.

The Behavior Perspective

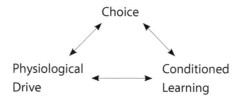

In Mr. R's case, he denies the use of any illicit substances and has no evidence of primary sleep or sexual disorders. He describes a life-long struggle with obesity and eating, but whether this represents a combination of disordered *choice,* physiologic *drive*, and conditioned *learning* emblematic of a disorder of behavior would be pure speculation. Thus, although Mr. R is obese, it is unclear if he has disordered eating behaviors, which would be important to address in long-term treatment. (Not all cases of obesity are due to behavioral disorders.) Mr. R had been in group therapy focused on helping him control the eating behaviors. He had never been in individual treatment focusing on his low mood. In general, Mr. R's problem does not seem to be one where repetition of a behavior is the central feature. Although the behavior perspective may be relevant to his obesity, a condition for which he wants help, it is not clear at this time that his eating is in any way central to understanding or treating his current psychiatric condition. The problem with which he presents now is not one of disordered eating—something he *does*—but disordered affect.

Our understanding of Mr. R, thus far, is that he is someone who has experienced many challenging circumstances in his life, including his mother's premature, sudden death, rejection by his father in adolescence, the abrupt dissolution of his long-term relationship with his fiancée, illness and death of other loved ones, and criminal charges against a family member. He has usually adapted successfully to past stressors but has had more trouble coping recently. We have concluded that the dimensional and behavior perspectives are not playing central roles in his current mood presentation. We can construct a meaningful narrative to explain his mood disorder as arising from his life circumstances, an explanation that we immediately understand as plausible, for which we have empathy, and for which psychotherapy is the recommended treatment. However, we have not yet concluded whether the life-story perspective is the best way to understand the origin of Mr. R's disordered affect.

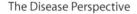

The Disease Perspective

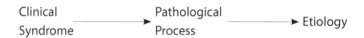

Clinical Syndrome → Pathological Process → Etiology

Disease-reasoning begins with the identification of a syndrome, so the first thing we want to know is whether Mr. R's illness has the form of a syndrome: a cluster of symptoms that occur together, run a course together, and respond to treatment together. Mr. R's current psychiatric condition fits well with a clinical *syndrome*. It consists of an insidious, two-year decline in his mood, vital sense (sleep, appetite, energy/motivation, concentration), and self-attitude of unknown *etiology* and *pathology*. In looking at Mr. R's psychiatric syndrome from the disease perspective, we must consider whether or not the current symptoms represent a new theme, best explained as arising from abnormality in the structure or function of his brain that has been thrust upon him (something that he *has*).

Mr. R presents with the twin problems of an insidious onset of depressive symptoms amid multiple life stressors. Before formulating his case, we will begin with a general discussion of the dilemmas that can occur when depressive symptoms arise, as they often do, in the setting of stressful life events. As mentioned previously, we often draw on story-telling to help understand changes that occur in our mental life and behavior following stressful life events. However, not every story we tell may be true. When patients—like Mr. R—or their physicians invoke meaningful explanations to understand new symptoms that can also be caused by a disease process, they risk falling into a trap. This is what we have called *the trap of meaning*, that is, finding an explanation that seems meaningful and adopting it as causal.[1] Meaningful explanations can obscure the true nature and origin of a patient's suffering. This misunderstanding of a patient's symptoms can contribute to multiyear delays in the diagnosis and treatment of depression,[2] at the risk of life-altering consequences, including suicide, at times.

When a patient like Mr. R presents to his physician with meaningful explanations for behavior and feelings, the physician is likely to accept these meaningful explanations at face value as the cause of the patient's behavior and feelings and, consequently, he or she may not initiate appropriate treatment. Fortunately in Mr. R's case, his physician recognized the syndrome of depression and started him on a trial of paroxetine; however, Mr. R—not considering his symptoms to be due to a depressive disorder—did not initiate a conversation with his physician about the adequacy of his dose, nor did his physician prescribe a higher dose (perhaps due to being "partially" caught in the trap of meaning).

We conclude that Mr. R's current condition is best thought of as a disease—major depression—whose pathologic etiology and mechanism remain to be elucidated, although Mr. R was initially skeptical of this formulation. Using the disease perspective's reasoning, appropriate pharmacotherapy is an indicated treatment for Mr. R, an intervention to which he agreed but for which he held little hope. The existing evidence is clear that combination treatment of antidepressant medication with specific psychotherapy is most likely to lead to remission of depression.[3] We do not reject the role of the life-story perspective in understanding his present condition—recognizing the role that psychotherapy can play in improve-ment in depressive symptoms—nor do we dismiss the role of psycho-therapy as a treatment for major depression.[4] But neither do we attribute his depressive symptoms solely to the multiple personal losses he has *en-countered*. Rather, we consider these symptoms as arising from the inter-action of an unknown pathologic process in Mr. R's brain provoked for the first time in his life by stressful occurrences, something Mr. R *has*. Intervening quickly to treat a first episode of a mood disorder provoked by psychosocial stressors can prevent a malignant progression of the de-pressive disorder.[5] Once the depression is treated, he may be ready to en-gage in psychotherapy to address other life-story and behavioral issues, such as his lifelong struggle with his weight. The application of the *Per-spectives* approach to Mr. R's case enables us both to understand him better and to make his treatment more whole.

Case Conclusion

Mr. R tolerated, but did not respond to, a long trial of 20 mg paroxetine daily. Therefore, Dr. Cohen recommends an increase in the daily dose to 40 mg, which Mr. R tolerates well. Mr. R gradually improves and, after six weeks on 40 mg paroxetine daily, his mood returns to its usual level of cheer. He is surprised and delighted by this response to an adjustment in dose. Mr. R begins to clean up his home, resumes his master's program studies, and begins teaching a new Sunday school class. Although indi-vidual psychotherapy is offered, he participates in only two sessions. With pharmacotherapy and this brief psychotherapy, he is able to move on from past stresses and face the ongoing issues with his usual strength and poise. Although some of his sadness may have been due to life events, the depressive syndrome with which he presented seems to have been primar-ily due to the disease of depression, which was treated successfully with an antidepressant. Mr. R's experience is not unlike the experiences of many other patients who live for years with an incorrect understanding of the cause of their illness, stuck in a trap of meaning until their symp-toms become overwhelming or seriously affect functioning—or until oth-ers close to them intervene to help them access appropriate care. Not unexpectedly, such patients are often surprised, as Mr. R was, when their behavior changes and symptoms remit after proper treatment, while the life circumstances they considered to be the cause of their problems stay the same.

Summary Points

1 Current depressive symptoms in the setting of stress need to be considered in the context of the patient's past responses to stressful situations

2 Syndromic patterns (such as the one of major depressive disorder seen here) that represent a departure from the usual theme of a person's life are better understood as diseases

3 Beware the trap of meaning

A Matriarch with Memory and Mood Problems

Managing Diagnostic Dilemmas

D r. Lauder, a neuropsychiatrist, is asked to see Ms. S, a 65-year-old woman referred by her primary-care physician, Dr. Green, for an evaluation of depressed mood of three to four months' duration, and memory loss of one year's duration. Ms. S is accompanied by her husband.

(Dr. Lauder's comments are printed in *italics*.)

Good morning, Ms. S. Dr. Green asked me to see you. I've reviewed her referral notes, but I'd like to hear in your own words why you're here today.

I've been having such memory troubles. I'm forever forgetting where I put things, and my husband tells me I'm repeating myself. Mom got Alzheimer's when she was just my age, and I'm worried that I've got it too. I knew it would come to this. I've worried my whole life that I'd end up like my mother.

Mr. S, would you like to add anything to what your wife has told me?

Well, yes. She's usually such an outgoing and social person. But lately, she's been keeping to herself, and most mornings I wake up to find her crying to herself.

When did you first notice these changes?

I'd say three to four months ago, at least. She seems to be slowly getting worse.

Now, Ms. S, I'd like to start with your family history. Has anyone else in your family had psychiatric conditions?

Before she got Alzheimer's, Mom was a big worrier, but she never saw anybody for that. My parents separated when I was young, so I don't know much about what went on with my father. I know he saw someone for depression after his stroke. He was well into his 70s. I don't know what kind of medicine they gave him, but whatever it was, it helped a lot.

Are they still alive?

No, they've both passed now.

How was their health otherwise?

Mom was always fine, except for the worrying, before the Alzheimer's. I know my father had high blood pressure and cholesterol problems, but—besides that and the stroke—nothing else. I guess that's enough.

Any psychiatric conditions in your extended family—anybody else with Alzheimer's?

Nothing. Nobody else has it, as far as I know.

Can you tell me more about your mother's Alzheimer's?

Well, let's see . . . Mom started having problems when she was in her early 60s. By the time she was 65, she had to go into a home. That was hard on me. I'm an only child, and we were really close. Mom lingered for almost ten years before she passed.

How long ago was that?

It's coming up on twenty years ago now. I was 45 when she passed. . . . Toward the end, I couldn't stand to go visit her there. She didn't even know it was me. I still went anyway. It seemed like the right thing to do.

That must have been very difficult. Do you and your husband have any children?

Yes, two grown daughters and five grandchildren. They're a joy.

How old are your daughters?

Chrissie's 40 and Linda's 35. Chrissie takes after my mother, with all the worrying. And that's gotten worse now that she has kids. But she's never gone to see anyone either. They're both stubborn as mules, my mother and Chrissie.

And Linda?

Oh, she's fine. She just had her second baby and she's calm as can be.

(Ms. S is asked about and denies any problems during gestation, infancy, and childhood.)

Where did you go to school?

I went to a Quaker school, even though we weren't Quakers. I wasn't much of a student, though. I was more interested in boys. I was named Miss Congeniality at graduation.

You must have been fairly outgoing?

Oh, yes, I've always had a lot of friends.

What did you do for a living?

I was a secretary on Capitol Hill for nearly thirty-five years. I loved my job. But when the Senator retired two years ago, so did I. Now I get to spend more time with my grandchildren.

Do you enjoy that?

Yes, I really do. But it seems like I'm slowing down. I just don't seem to have the energy that I used to, which makes it tough to keep up with them.

And how long have you and your husband been married?

We've been together for forty years. I love him very much, but I tell you, we've had our differences at times. Dr. Green sent us to a marriage counselor about five years ago to help us make peace. We saw the counselor two or three times, and things are better now.

I'm glad to hear that you were able to work things out. What type of marital problems were you having?

My husband was getting on my nerves. He's more particular about a lot of things than I am, and he likes things just so.

Can you give me an example?

Well, let's see . . . for instance, he's a morning person, and I'm not. If I didn't get up by 8:00 on weekends, he'd get upset that I was wasting our day away. When we started to fight, I thought about leaving him. The counselor helped us learn to pick our battles, and we hardly bicker at all anymore.

Mr. S, do you have anything to add here?

Well, I agree that things got better after we went to counseling, but I still wish she would be more orderly. She used to tidy up after herself, but for the last couple of years, she doesn't put anything away after she takes it out, and she's forever starting projects that she never finishes. She was never this bad.

Are you saying her forgetfulness may have started more than a year ago?

Well, I never thought of it that way. I thought it had to do with retiring from her job and not having that routine she'd had for all those years . . .

I am going to switch topics. Ms. S, do you drink or smoke?

I don't smoke. I have a glass of wine with dinner a couple of times a week. I've never been much of a drinker, really.

Do you have any medical problems?

Yes, my cholesterol is slightly elevated. Dr. Green recently started me on rosuvastatin.

Any other medical problems?

She has also told me that I have irritable bowel syndrome because my bowel movements alternate from hard to really loose. My colonoscopy last year was completely normal, though.

Do you take any medications other than the rosuvastatin?

Yes, I take citalopram 20 mg every day, zopli-something . . .

Zolpidem?

Yes, that's it, 5 mg at night, and diazepam 2 mg a day when I need it for my nerves. Dr. Green gives them all to me. But I only take the diazepam once or twice a week when my anxiety gets the better of me.

I'm going to change topics once again. Ms. S, can you tell me about what you're usually like as a person and what your interests are?

Sure. I'm usually a very cheerful and friendly person, although my husband says I worry too much, and I guess I do. We go for walks every day with our dogs. And I also take care of our grandbabies, and I like to cook. Oh, and I love playing solitaire on my television.

Mr. S, is that how you would describe your wife?

Well, she is very outgoing, and does get along with most everybody. She's got a big heart and has an artistic side. She can be a little too sensitive, I think.

What do you mean?

Well, she's always the first one in the family to cry during a sad movie. And she's also a bit of a spitfire. She'll lose her temper if things don't go her way. Like when I tell her she needs to clean up after herself . . .

Ms. S, have you ever experienced any emotional problems prior to your current difficulties?

No, I wouldn't say so. I've always worried about things more than my husband, but I never felt that kept me from doing what I needed to get done.

Have you ever seen a psychiatrist or psychologist prior to today?

No, only the marriage counselor.

Let's return to the recent difficulties that you have been having, Ms. S. When did you first develop difficulties with your memory?

Now, I'm not entirely sure. I would say at least a year ago, but I've noticed it's gotten much worse in the last couple of months. Early on, I had problems keeping track of where I was putting things, you know, around the house. Once, I forgot my purse at the grocery store check-out, which was a real scare. Lately, it's getting harder to remember what day it is or appointments I've made. I now have to carry a calendar with me at all times so that I can keep track of everything.

Have you gotten lost or had any accidents around the house?

No, not yet, but I tell you, this is a big fear of mine. I'm still driving but I've considered stopping.

Do you ever notice any problems finding words when you are speaking?

Yes. That's a big one. I feel like a word is caught on the tip of my tongue. Usually I can get it out with help from my husband.

Ms. S, are you able to care for yourself and take care of routine household chores, like paying the bills, or do you require help?

Well, I'm pretty good at taking care of myself. And I can still cook all our meals, but my husband now does the shopping. We've had a maid service for years, so I haven't cleaned the house myself in a while. And my husband's always managed our money and paid the bills.

Mr. S, do you agree with what your wife has told me about her memory problems?

Yes, we've been lucky that there haven't been any accidents around the house or while she's driving. We count our blessings for that every day.

Thank you. Now, Ms. S, I'd like to ask you about your mood of late. How has your mood been recently?

I really haven't been myself. It's hard to put how I'm feeling into words, but I just don't have my usual pep. And I'm not as interested in things as I used to be.

Have you been feeling sad?

Yes, I must say I have. Sometimes it just overcomes me and I can't fight back the tears. I'm so worried that I have dementia. I wish God would just take me before I become a burden to my husband.

I'm so sorry you feel that way. Have you been having any thoughts of taking your life?

Oh, no! I would never take my own life. I wouldn't want to hurt my family.

I see from your records that Dr. Green started you on citalopram, zolpidem, and diazepam about six weeks ago. Have you noticed any improvement in any of your symptoms with these medications?

No, I haven't. If anything, I think my memory is worse, and the diarrhea's been terrible.

Have you had any other side effects?

No, just the memory and diarrhea.

Have you been able to identify any triggers that seemed to bring about your recent difficulties?

My mood went down after I started to have these problems with my memory. I don't think I'd be depressed at all if I didn't have these memory problems. Who wouldn't be depressed if they had Alzheimer's?

Mr. S, do you have anything to add to what your wife has told me about her recent mood changes?

I notice that she isn't sleeping like she used to. She seems to toss and turn a good hour or two each night. She's also mentioned to me that she wakes up much earlier than she wants to, around 5 or 6, and then she usually can't fall back to sleep and is tired the rest of the day. She also can have brief spells in which she becomes testy with me, but it never gets physical. As I mentioned earlier, she's also been keeping to herself more. She just recently canceled two trips with our family, and she refuses to meet her friends for lunch anymore.

How's her appetite?

That's never been big, but it's definitely gotten worse recently. She's lost almost 15 pounds in the last two months.

MSE: Ms. S is an alert, well-groomed woman who appears younger than her stated age. She engages well during the assessment but appears anxious. Ms. S has mild psychomotor agitation characterized by wringing of her hands and shaking of her legs up and down while sitting. She becomes tearful when asked questions about her memory. She demonstrates good eye contact. Her comprehension is good. Her speech is slightly slow, with decreased volume, but her associations are intact. Ms. S makes one paraphasic error, substituting *television* for *computer.* No other language errors are observed. She reports her mood as "not good," and her mood is assessed as sad and anxious. Ms. S describes extreme worry about having dementia like her mother did. Ms. S also reports a great fear that she will "linger" in a nursing home like her mother did. Ms. S's vital sense and self-attitude are diminished. She feels that she is no longer able to be a good wife and is hopeless about the future. Ms. S reports passive death wishes, but denies thoughts of suicide and homicide. There are no delusions, hallucinations, obsessions, compulsions, panic attacks, or phobias. Ms. S scores 22/30 on the MMSE: she misses 2 points on orientation, 4 on attention, and 2 on recall. When asked to name as many four-legged animals as possible in 30 seconds, she names similar animals together and, with this strategy, is able to name six animals, which is a bit below normal. Her vocabulary and comprehension, as well as descriptive abilities, exhibited during the interview support an assessment of baseline normal intelligence. Ms. S's insight is limited in that she expresses understanding that her memory and mood are not normal, but does not have a full understanding of the extent of her problems. Ms. S is willing to come for a psychiatric evaluation of her mood and memory disturbances. Further, she has been taking the medications prescribed by Dr. Green, all of which suggests that her judgment is intact. A neurologic exam is normal with no evidence of Parkinsonism or focal deficits. Ms. S's gait is slow but otherwise normal.

Case Discussion

Steps 2–4: History, MSE, and Collateral Informants

Ms. S is a 65-year-old woman who presents for an evaluation of two problems: progressive memory difficulties and recent mood changes. She has a family history of Alzheimer disease (AD) in her mother and depression following a stroke in her father. Ms. S is a high school graduate who held a steady job as a secretary until she retired two years ago. She has been married for forty years. She and her husband have had a stable relationship, except for brief marital difficulties several years ago that resolved with the help of a counselor. Ms. S has a close relationship with her children and grandchildren.

Ms. S and her husband noticed that her memory began to decline approximately one year ago. Her cognitive disturbances are characterized by short-term memory loss (e.g., misplacing items around the house and forgetting appointments), impaired executive functioning (e.g., disorganization, impaired planning), and occasional language difficulties (e.g., trouble with word-finding). Ms. S's ability to perform basic activities of daily living is largely preserved, although she is less able to do instrumental activities, such as shopping. The memory loss has accelerated in the prior two to three months in the setting of depressive symptoms including pervasive sad-to-irritable mood, insomnia with early morning awakening, poor appetite with a 15-pound weight loss, anhedonia, fatigue, increased memory loss, and feeling she is becoming a burden. Ms. S is also experiencing anxiety, fearing the prognosis of her memory complaints. Despite the initiation of citalopram one month ago, she has had little relief from her recent mood disturbances. The MSE confirms Ms. S's reported mood disturbances including sad and anxious mood, decreased vital sense, and diminished self-attitude. The MMSE reveals impairments in orientation, attention, and short-term recall. Further, Ms. S is noted to have impaired executive functioning. Her language is grossly intact, although she made one paraphasic error during the assessment.

Step 5: Consideration from Each Perspective

The Life-Story Perspective

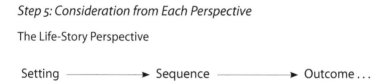

Ms. S was in her usual state of health until approximately one year ago, when she first developed memory difficulties. Ms. S and her husband observed her mood decline several months after the onset of her memory problems. Neither Ms. S nor her husband recalls any particularly stressful life event that might have contributed to her recent memory or mood symptoms, other than the fact that years ago she saw her mother's deterioration and death from dementia. She appears very upset that she may develop and die from the same disease as her mother. Ms. S, however, does think her recent anxiety and sadness are due to her concern—given her mother's dementia—about the possible significance of her own memory loss. We, too, might be inclined to make such a connection. Although such an explanation makes sense temporally, is intuitive, and may indeed be the case, the mood change and its associated symptoms, such as impaired self-attitude and early morning awakening, appear to represent a recognizable syndrome (to be discussed when we consider the disease perspective). Thus, the stereotypical form of the clinical syndrome with which she presents cannot be explained fully by Ms. S's life story. Further, her mood state seems to be in excess of the stressor since, despite cognitive symptoms, it has not been a foregone conclusion that she has dementia or AD, as she has not yet been evaluated. And, although Ms. S fears that her own cognitive difficulties could represent a dementia such as her mother had, the cognitive symptoms themselves are hard to attribute entirely to that fear.

The Dimensional Perspective

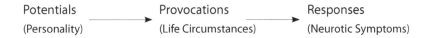

Potentials   →   Provocations   →   Responses

(Personality)   (Life Circumstances)   (Neurotic Symptoms)

Ms. S appears to be of average intelligence. Based on the history, she is typically outgoing, sociable, and usually quite cheerful, although inclined to worry. While this tendency to worry is one dimension associated with introversion, someone who is described as "the life of the party" is more likely to rest on the extraverted side of the introversion-extraversion dimension. Looking at the instability–great stability dimension, Ms. S appears to be a sensitive person who is easily angered at times but has been able to maintain stable and close long-term relationships with her husband and children, except for a brief period of marital discord several years ago. Further, she has been employed throughout her adult life without reported interpersonal difficulties in the workplace. Although she does not lie on an extreme on the instability–great stability dimension, she appears to rest slightly on the instability side of this dimension. Because she does not rest on an extreme of either dimension, we conclude that cognitive or mood dimensional vulnerability is insufficient to explain fully the origin of her current difficulties. Therefore, we do not see Ms. S's present condition arising primarily from who she *is* as a person. Nevertheless, it is important to recognize that her recent angst surrounding her health is likely influenced by her temperamental predisposition to worry.

The Behavior Perspective

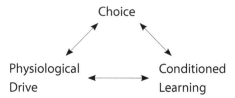

Ms. S has no history of abnormal behaviors (e.g., illicit substance use, eating, sexual) that can account for her memory and mood symptoms. Therefore, we conclude that Ms. S's presentation cannot be attributed to problematic, repetitive behaviors.

The Disease Perspective

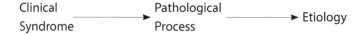

Ms. S has experienced progressive decline in memory over the last year, accompanied by a number of depressive symptoms as well as prominent anxiety. Based on Dr. Lauder's assessment, Ms. S demonstrates cognitive dysfunction marked by impaired short-term memory and executive dysfunction. She also displays inattention, has reduced verbal fluency, and makes a notable paraphasic error. Her other cognitive domains appear to be intact, although more complete cognitive testing might reveal more subtle impairments. Her daily functioning appears to be somewhat impaired at this time (e.g., "I'm forever forgetting where I put things" and "my husband now does the shopping"). Therefore, Ms. S's presentation takes the form of a global cognitive decline with functional impact occurring in the absence of delirium. She meets *DSM* criteria for dementia, a recognizable syndrome even though the cognitive decline and functional impairment are mild. The cause of this condition is uncertain. Since Ms. S's memory loss has accelerated in the setting of recent mood symptoms (see below), this raises the possibility that depression is producing at least part of the cognitive disturbance ("Dementia of Depression"). Further, Ms. S reports that her memory worsened following initiation of the current psychotropic regimen. Thus, dementia secondary to the effects from one or more medications, in particular the sedatives, is included in the differential diagnosis. Next, other causes of dementia need to be ruled out. A partial list of such conditions includes: brain vascular disease (e.g., stroke, white matter disease), hypothyroidism, diabetes, and many others. However, in light of the family history, AD cannot be ruled out. For further discussion of the evaluation of dementia refer to *Practical Dementia Care*.[1]

In regard to her mood symptoms, Ms. S describes a low, anxious, and irritable mood, with insomnia, poor appetite, fatigue, and diminished self-worth. Ms. S therefore currently exhibits all aspects of a major depressive episode with onset in later life, a recognizable syndrome. Although some may argue that her prominent anxiety merits an additional diagnosis of an anxiety disorder, using Occam's razor, we consider her anxiety as a manifestation of the major depressive episode, since anxiety symptoms are common in late-life depression. While later life onset is unusual for major depressive disorder it is possible that this is the cause of her mood disturbance. There is no history of mania to warrant a diagnosis of bipolar disorder. Finally, since later onset major depression, compared to early onset, is more likely to be caused by brain diseases, and is occurring in the context of a dementia, other causes of depression need to be ruled out, such as the ones discussed above that might also be causing dementia.

We have used the disease perspective to identify Ms. S's illness as syndromic in nature, characterized by a cluster of cognitive and mood symptoms. Although these take the form of two syndromes, one cognitive (dementia) and one mood (major depressive episode), because the disease perspective asks whether the clinical syndrome arises from abnormality in the structure or function of the brain, it is possible that both syndromes arise from the same pathology and etiology. Thus, the diagnostic evaluation for the cause of dementia is a diagnostic evaluation for the cause of the depressive episode, at least partly so. Since depression is often associated with AD, this strengthens the likelihood that she is in the early stages of this progressive neurodegenerative disease, which has caused both the depressive episode and the dementia.

Steps 6 and 7: Formulation and Treatment Plan

Ms. S's case presents a diagnostic dilemma. She is a generally stable, extraverted woman who presents with both cognitive and mood symptoms and has witnessed her mother's cognitive decline from dementia. By applying the *Perspectives* approach we are able to consider the likelihood that Ms. S's cognitive and/or mood symptoms have arisen from her life story (what she has *encountered*), personality (who she *is*), behavior (what she *does*), or disease (what she *has*). Given the presence of recognizable syndromes, as well as the well-known association of dementia with depression in this age group, we conclude that Ms. S's condition is the result of a brain disease. The etiologic mechanism through which late-life brain disease causes conditions such as this, especially major depression, is unknown. It is presumed to arise from an undetectable, at present, alteration in brain structure/function. A trial of another antidepressant medication for the depressive episode, combined with ongoing follow-up in the setting of a psychotherapeutic relationship with her psychiatrist, is the recommended treatment. Nevertheless, we remain suspicious that she may be in early stages of AD, for which she will need additional testing, individual supportive psychotherapy, and close monitoring.

This kind of systematic approach to Ms. S's history, MSE, and formulation is not only helpful in reaching the treatment recommendation, but also contributes to our understanding of Ms. S as a whole, which will then inform her psychotherapy treatment. Although Ms. S's presentation of mood and cognitive symptoms seems largely explained by the disease perspective, this perspective alone does not capture the full breadth of Ms. S's distress. Her symptoms occur against the background of a mildly anxious and extraverted person. Ms. S has long had a concern that she will develop progressive dementia and spend her final years in a nursing home like her mother. In the setting of uncertainty about her underlying diagnosis, Ms. S has experienced escalation of longstanding fears about her cognition. Therefore, these additional aspects of her recent distress may be better understood by combining insights from the life-story and dimensional perspectives. Out of this *Perspectives*-based formulation, a comprehensive treatment for Ms. S will include pharmacotherapy as well as individual psychotherapy aimed at optimizing her quality of life and offering her support and guidance regarding her fears about her health and dying.

Case Conclusion

Given Ms. S's history and MSE, Dr. Lauder orders serum, urine, neuropsychological, and brain imaging studies. Urine studies are normal. Serum studies reveal normal complete blood count, metabolic panel, thyroid panel, and vitamin B_{12} and serum folate levels. Neuropsychological testing reveals global cognitive impairment characterized by impaired short-term memory, executive functioning, visual learning, visuospatial planning and organization, and object-naming, confirming the initial impression of dementia. A brain MRI reveals no obvious causes of her condition, as there is no evidence of infarcts, significant white matter change, or other abnormalities. A major part of the initial treatment plan is to treat the depression and remove medications that may be affecting her cognition.

To address the depression, over a three-month period, Dr. Lauder titrates the mirtazapine to 30 mg nightly, while she concurrently tapers and eventually discontinues the diazepam, in addition to engaging Ms. S in individual psychotherapy. Ms. S's mood returns to normal and she reports feeling much better physically and not worrying much about her memory loss. Her diarrhea resolves, she gains back 10 pounds, and she resumes her usual hobbies, including regularly meeting her friends for lunch.

Unfortunately, Ms. S's cognitive impairment persists, and over the course of the following year, worsens. Her husband later reports that she is beginning to become confused when driving and has left a burner lit on the stove, despite his close supervision. Given the progressive nature of the decline, despite successful treatment of depression, Dr. Lauder revises Ms. S's diagnosis to dementia due to AD with associated depression and recommends that Ms. S's driving privileges be removed. Dr. Lauder then begins to develop and implement a tailored program of dementia care[1] in conjunction with a local memory center, including initiation of a cholinesterase inhibitor. She advises the family that Ms. S should have continual supervision, which Mr. S provides with support from their children and a privately hired home health aide. In light of this revised diagnosis and the growing dependence on her husband, Ms. S experiences a recurrence of anxiety and fear, although not a full major depressive episode. Dr. Lauder formulates these symptoms using a life-story approach and begins to see Ms. S and her husband together to develop strategies to maximize Ms. S's quality of life, combat her demoralization caused by the diagnosis of Alzheimer dementia, and help them prepare for the next stages of her disease.

Summary Points

1   A patient's psychiatric condition is shaped by a combination of her unique life story and temperamental strengths and vulnerabilities, even when the patient suffers from brain disease

2   A strong therapeutic relationship helps a patient and family manage and prepare for different phases of illness

3   Syndromic patterns (such as dementia and major depressive episode) that represent a departure from the usual theme of a person's life are better understood as diseases

An Executive with Health Worries

Dimension or Disease?

Agynecologic (gyn) nurse practitioner refers Ms. B, a 46-year-old woman, to Dr. Hudson for an outpatient psychiatric evaluation of persistent intractable health worries. With Ms. B's permission, her nurse practitioner calls Dr. Hudson to share her perspective on the patient.

(Dr. Hudson's comments are printed in *italics*.)

Thanks for referring Ms. B, and I'm glad we can talk before I see her.

I'm so relieved you can see her. She really needs help. She's not been herself for months. She's usually a very rational and stable person. But over the past six months, she's become crazy with worry about her health, which, I assure you, is 100% fine. It started when she thought she felt a lump in her breast, and so I ordered a mammogram, which was thankfully negative. But since then, she's been calling the office constantly with worries about more lumps, all of which have turned out to be nothing. I end up spending more time trying to calm her down than I do examining her. But nothing I say seems to allay her fears.

Has she ever had any psychiatric condition like this before that you know of?

I don't think so. Like I said, she's always seemed very stable and I've known her for over ten years. Her internist recently recommended she start an SSRI, but I'm not sure if she even ever tried it. Before this, I've never seen any sign of anxiety or depression.

Okay. Anything else that you think I should know before meeting her? Is she taking any other medications?

Just the same oral contraceptive she's been on for years: low dose norethindrone-ethinyl estradiol. She has no medical problems at all. Last time she was here she asked if I knew any good cardiologists because her blood pressure was 135/85 and she was worried about having heart disease. That was the first time I'd heard her worry about anything other than cancer.

Well, I look forward to meeting her and thanks again for the referral. I'll be back in contact, with her permission, after the evaluation.

(Dr. Hudson greets Ms. B and welcomes her into his office.)

Welcome, Ms. B. It's nice to meet you. I spoke with your gyn. She said she thought you hadn't seen a psychiatrist before.

Yes, this is the last place I ever thought I'd be.

Let's begin by talking a little about what led you to come here today.

Really, this whole year has been a disaster. First it was my neck, then the breast stuff, and now I'm all worked up about this thing on my hand. See this here, on the left side? It's been bothering me for a month. I finally got in to see my dermatologist yesterday, and he said it was just a freckle, but I'm not convinced. I know it sounds crazy, and maybe it is.

I can see you're still worried. We'll spend most of our time today talking about these worries, but I'd like to first learn more about you and your background. Can you tell me about your family?

There's not that much to tell. Mom stayed at home with us 'til George, my youngest brother, finished high school, and then she started working at the library downtown. She's still there part time.

And your dad?

We've never been that close, especially since he and mom separated about ten years ago, when she found out he was having an affair. I really haven't seen him much since, which is fine with me. He was always a super angry guy—I never knew about what—and drank a lot of liquor. He got nastier and nastier as he got older; just wanted to stay by himself and not be bothered by any of us. Mom was a saint to put up with him as long as she did.

(Ms. B is asked about her parents' health and states that they're both in good health.)

Have your father or mother ever had psychiatric treatment?

Well, Dad *should* have. But, of course, he never saw anyone. Mom's always been fine, though I think she takes some kind of pill for her nerves every once in a while. She's become more of a worrier in her old age.

Did your parents tend to get along during your childhood?

No. They were always fighting. They still do when he comes back for Christmas and Easter. I can't believe she lets him back in the house after the things he did.

You mean the affair?

Well, there's that. But there were also a couple of times when he hit her, never that bad—no bruising or broken bones, I mean. But still. But I never saw her be scared of him. She's a strong woman.

What about you. Were you scared? Did he ever hit you?

No, he never hit us kids, but we were definitely scared of him. We never knew when he was going to go off.

You mentioned your brothers. Any sisters?

No, it's just the three of us. George's the youngest—he's 40, I'm the oldest, and Charlie's in the middle at 43.

How are they doing?

They're pretty good. George used to smoke a lot of pot but he quit before he got married. They just had their first—a cute baby boy. Charlie's divorced and remarried. Charlie never smoked pot or drank, but he went through some rough times after his divorce. I know he saw someone for depression for a while. He tried some kind of antidepressant but he didn't like the side effects, I think. Charlie's kind of like me in a lot of ways. We're both extremely organized, very hard working. He owns his own business, building luxury boats.

And tell me about your extended family—anyone you know of who has had any psychological problems or any trouble with alcohol or drugs?

My grandfather—my dad's dad—tried to OD on pills when he was in his 70s. He went to a hospital after that for a few months. He was like my dad—angry a lot. Drank a lot of whiskey, too. My mom's dad also drank a lot, though I remember him as more of a happy, social beer drinker.

Any suicides anywhere in the family?

No.

(Ms. B denies any problems during gestation, infancy, or early childhood.)

Tell me about your school years and how you liked school.

School was great. I was a good student; got mostly Bs. We moved to Syracuse when I was 13, which wasn't easy, but I ended up making friends pretty fast.

You mentioned that your dad and one of your brothers had a drinking problem. Did you do any drinking in high school?

Just a little bit, on weekends, at parties. I don't have much of a tolerance for alcohol. At our high school, pot was more popular, and I did smoke a little one summer with my girlfriends. But once school started again we started hanging out with other people and I never smoked again. At college, I drank even less than in high school—maybe two beers on the weekend if I went to a party.

Did you date in high school?

I had a steady boyfriend from tenth grade 'til we graduated high school.

Were you sexually active?

No, just some making out, nothing else. My husband, Brian, is the only one I've been with, and even with him it wasn't until we got engaged that we first slept together.

And where did you and Brian meet?

We both went to Syracuse. It's a real party school, and I think we must have been the only ones who were actually going to class. Plus, we were both working full time and living with our parents. He was in my biology lab group freshman year and we studied together. We were engaged by our junior year and got married right after graduation. We've been together ever since. We've made a good life for ourselves. We bought a lake house about fifteen years ago. I planned out a timetable for paying off both mortgages, which we just did last year, a year ahead of schedule.

And what does your husband think about your illness?

He really doesn't know what to think. At first, of course, he was worried about my physical health, but at this point he's starting to think I'm a little nuts. And I don't blame him.

How's your sexual relationship?

Well, we haven't had sex at all since I've been sick. But, before then, it wasn't that good either. Since we've had kids, we only have sex once a month, at most. And he's always the one who initiates it. I guess neither of us has much of a sex drive, so it works out okay.

When did you begin having children?

Around the time we got the lake house. Cody's 15 and Justin's 16. They're both great kids. Justin's second grade teacher thought he might have ADD and so his pediatrician prescribed some kind of stimulant medication, but Justin never liked it. I tried some too, out of curiosity—it just made me feel wound up.

What was the name of that medication?

They were the generic kind . . . methylphenidate.

I have a few more questions before we talk about how you've been doing lately. Tell me about the jobs you've had.

Well, I've been at the same place since college. It's just a little, local business. Thank God we've never been bought out by one of the national firms. I don't like change.

Is it stressful at all?

Not usually. I actually love my work. I've been promoted three times and I'm now a manager. Sometimes a crisis develops that I have to respond to, which can be a little stressful. To be honest, though, I'm more bored than stressed there. But I've been keeping busy with other things. Like we just finished redecorating the lake house and we're now remodeling the basement. And I'm doing some part-time work for my brother's business. If that takes off, I may eventually leave my regular job. It depends a lot on the economy, though. I'm not one to rush into anything.

You seem to know yourself pretty well. Your gyn said she's known you for a long time and that you're a pretty stable and together person. How would you describe yourself, before things started changing this past year?

Well, I've always been highly organized and very goal-driven. Sometimes I'll go on a mission, cleaning the house from top to bottom, or, like when we were looking to buy the lake house, researching every single house on the market. My husband says I'm like a dog with a bone. I get hooked on a project and I can't think of anything else until it's done. It drives him crazy. Plus I never ask for help. I think I just try never to show any weakness, as a rule. With friends, I tend to be a problem-solver and keep things pretty upbeat, though I do that less now, since I've been so worried about my health.

Do you have close friends?

I get along with everyone, but I tend to spend more time with family than friends. My husband's really my closest friend.

Are you someone who tends to doubt yourself?

Not really. I don't much second-guess myself. I'm pretty confident in my decisions, once I make my mind up.

Is that hard for you?

Well, I like to think things through first. I enjoy that. I don't like being impulsive. I like weighing the pros and cons and making sure I know what I'm getting into. I don't want to regret making a bad decision. I want to make sure it turns out the way I expect it to. I guess I'm a bit of a perfectionist that way.

Sounds like you're pretty self-reliant, too.

Yes, that bothers my husband a lot. He thinks I should consult him more, but really I'm much more particular than he is, and it's mostly my money. Financial independence has always been really important to me. I didn't want to be like my mother: dependent on a man.

Would you describe yourself as normally being an anxious person?

Not at all. I plan and think things through, but I don't tend to worry.

Has anyone ever described you as a dramatic person?

Nope. Most people describe me as calm.

What do you like to do for fun?

Like I said, I tend to take on projects, like getting the lake house, doing renovations, things like that. That's fun for me. I don't have the patience for knitting and I wouldn't want to join a book club or anything like that. I like big, long-term projects that I can tackle on my own.

I'd like to switch gears a bit now and get back to what brought you here today. Have you ever had worries about your health like this before?

No. Never.

Or any times when you felt sad or down most of the time?

Well, when I was in high school, there were times when I felt down, but I always bounced back pretty quickly. My mom used to call them my sad phases.

How long did these phases last?

Just a couple of weeks at most. And they didn't happen a lot—maybe three or four times a year. It was usually at the end of each quarter grading period, when a lot of papers and projects were due.

What were those times like?

I don't remember a lot about them. I think I had trouble sleeping. I'd stay up worrying about all the stuff I needed to get done. I didn't eat as much. I'd get upset about things more easily and cry, which wasn't like me.

Did you ever think about suicide during these times?

No. I'd never heard of anyone doing that, except in books. I never thought about it.

Have you continued to have these times as an adult?

No, aside from being worried now, I've been fine.

(The patient is asked about and denies any symptoms of mania, panic disorder, and social phobias.)

I know that you have had a lot of worries lately about health concerns, which we'll talk about next. But aside from the concerns about breast and skin cancer, do you have any medical illnesses and are you taking any medications?

The only medicine I'm on now is the birth control pills, which are the same ones I've been taking since Cody was born.

I'd like to take a few minutes and ask you some questions about how you're feeling physically right now. Have you gained or lost any weight?

I've lost about 20 pounds since all of this started.

Any fatigue?

I've been feeling more and more tired over the past year. If anyone asks me how I feel, I now usually say, "Exhausted."

Any trouble breathing?

I feel like I'm always holding my breath, but when I realize that, I can breathe fine.

Any constipation or diarrhea?

I've had a little diarrhea lately—not really more often. I still just go once a day. It's now just a little looser than usual.

Any dizziness or lightheadedness?

No. Well, a little when I first get out of bed in the morning.

Any problems with your thyroid?

Not that I know of. I know I've asked my doctor to check this, since I've been so tired, and she said it was fine.

(Please note that Dr. Hudson performs a complete review of systems, but only the symptoms endorsed by Ms. B are included here.)

OK. Let's move on to when you last felt well, and what happened next.

Oh, boy! The last time I felt well was probably a year ago. As it started getting really cold, I started getting these aches in the middle of my neck, right here (the patient motions to the base of her skull). I tried taking aspirin, but it didn't help much. I started getting worried it might be a tumor, and what would happen to my boys if I was gone?

How was it that you went from noticing neck pain to fearing you had a tumor?

I don't know. That's just where my mind went. My neck hurt and—boom, boom—I thought I must have a tumor. My internist basically brushed me off.

What did he say?

Dr. K thought I'd just pulled something and it would go away. I insisted on an MRI, which he went along with. It turned out pretty much normal, although there was some very slight "disc bulging" in my neck, which he said was typical for someone my age. I was still convinced I had a tumor, so when the aches didn't go away in a couple of weeks I made an appointment with a neurologist. This was in January. The earliest she could see me was in four weeks, and those four weeks were pure agony. I was a basket case, worrying all the time about having some sort of spinal cancer. When the appointment finally came I got some relief. She examined me from head to toe and did another MRI, and this one was totally normal. They didn't even see the disc bulging this time! By that time, the pain had gone away and I could finally relax, and for a little while I was almost back to my old self. My friend at work told me that she was happy to see me joking around again, that I seemed less withdrawn.

Was there anything else going on in your life at the time that was especially stressful or difficult to deal with?

No, not really. Things with Brian and the boys were fine, and work was the same as always.

Did you know anyone who had a tumor or cancer of the spine?

Not the spine, but I do have a friend from college—Mary—whose cousin just died of ovarian cancer.

Have you had any worries about having ovarian cancer?

Sure, but I seem to worry about all sorts of things that I could have—anything I'm really aware of. Little things end up becoming major things with me. For a while I was up late every night looking up colon cancer on the Internet because I'd been constipated. Then, it was vulvar cancer because of what turned out to be an inflamed gland, then brain tumors because of headaches. Breast cancer was probably the worst. That started after Mary's cousin died. I'd always done my self-exams on the first day of my period, just like the doctor told me, and never noticed anything. But this past summer I thought I might have felt a lump in my left breast, which of course got me panicked. I was feeling for it every day, even going to the bathroom at work six or seven times a day to check it. I have to admit I still do an exam once a week, even though she told me not to. At my first appointment with her she couldn't feel it, but scheduled me for a mammogram later that week. When I got home I was so scared of what it might show that I called the center and pushed it back by two weeks. But then I was unbelievably worried about how, if it was cancer, it might metastasize and I'd better find out as soon as possible. I couldn't control my thoughts. The days after I got the mammogram were the worst, but thank God, the results came back negative. I could finally breathe again.

How long did that feeling last?

For about a month I was ok. Things got busy at work, and I started another big project at home, remodeling our basement. But that gnawing feeling that things aren't okay, that I'm not safe, came back. At my check-up with my internist I found out I have high blood pressure, and now I'm thinking I could be one of those people you hear about, you know, the woman who seemed fine but one day dropped dead of a heart attack while carrying her groceries up the driveway.

I'm sorry these thoughts, which are clearly so disturbing, keep coming back. Over this period, have you been on any medications for them?

Yes, but they've done more harm than good. I took alprazolam a few times last year when I was so worked up about the spine MRI. It wasn't much, maybe 0.5 mg, but I didn't want to get addicted. I've probably taken less than fifteen the whole year. This year, he tried me on sertraline, but I hated it. I couldn't sleep. I'd get nauseated and felt like I had the flu.

Do you remember what dose you were taking?

I started at 25 mg, but even when I tried cutting the pills into quarters, I still felt bad. After a few weeks I just stopped taking them. That was back in October.

Have you found anything, medication or otherwise, that's helped relieve your worries?

Most of the stuff I've read about on the Internet hasn't helped. Exercise has helped a little, and I try to eat foods that have high serotonin, but nothing works. I feel like my health is so poor—like I'm doomed to get sick.

It sounds like you're still thinking the problem is a physiological one—even though your doctors have said they can't find anything physically wrong.

Well, that's what I feel, but I'm here now because a part of me realizes I'm being irrational.

So you think there's a possibility that the problem is psychological?

I think I've gotten to that point. Yes.

How has your sleep been lately?

I don't think I've slept through the night for over a year. I wake up before dawn worrying about something and have a hard time going back to sleep. Almost every day I wake up at 4 in the morning and can't get back to sleep.

That sounds exhausting.

Like I said, I've been exhausted really, but I just keep forcing myself to do things. I think I'm mostly worn out from all the worrying. It really is hard to think about anything else. Maybe that's why I'm feeling bored at work. I don't know. I don't feel as motivated as I used to. I've even started making some little mistakes at work. Luckily I've caught them all, I think.

And you said you'd lost weight. Have you not had an appetite?

That's been terrible. Like I said, I've lost over 20 pounds this year.

What about your sex drive. Any recent change in your thoughts or interest?

That's always been pretty low. Even though we had more sex when we were first married, it's always been more important for my husband than me. Since we've had kids, I could really take it or leave it.

MSE: Ms. B is a slender woman. She is neatly dressed in clean, pressed slacks and a blouse. Her hair is well groomed and she is wearing minimal makeup. She has a normal gait and sits quietly with legs crossed. She has no hand tremors. She is cooperative and polite throughout the examination, but her eye contact is only fair, with frequent downward gaze. She is tearful at times, but also occasionally smiles and laughs. Her speech is unremarkable, with normal volume, rate, rhythm, intonation, fluency, and spontaneity, and with no evidence of a formal thought disorder. Ms. B reports her mood as sad, adding that she looks at everything in a sad way, though she denies anhedonia. She views herself as a good, successful person who loves her kids. When asked about the future she reports, "It's always looked bright, but now I'm worrying, where am I going to be in the future?" When asked directly whether she overall feels hopeful, however, she says that she does. She denies passive death wishes, and suicidal and homicidal thoughts. Ms. B believes that she's in poor health and that "it's only a matter of time" before she's diagnosed with a fatal illness. She describes heightened vigilance and sensitivity toward her perception of bodily changes. She is in a near-constant state of worry about her health and describes herself as being on "high alert." "I feel like I'm always holding my breath." Ms. B denies hallucinations, delusions, obsessions, and compulsions. Other than her fear of illness, she denies phobias. Her intelligence is judged to be above average based on her vocabulary. Her insight into her condition is good, as she realizes that her fear of having a morbid physical disease is irrational, given her health care providers' reassurances, and she is open to the possibility that her underlying problem may be psychological. Her judgment is impaired, as she seeks out medical specialists to evaluate a variety of somatic complaints that she perceives as having a physiological cause. Her MMSE score is 30/30.

The Discussion

Steps 2–4: History, MSE, and Collateral Information

Ms. B presents on recommendation by her gyn nurse practitioner after over a year of excessive worry about her health. She is temporarily reassured by negative test results about a particular source of worry, only to have a new worry surface for which she seeks objective reassurance. According to Ms. B and her nurse practitioner, she is usually a stable and rational woman who has achieved success in her educational, occupational, and family roles. She may have suffered from mild depressive episodes in adolescence, but has previously never sought any mental health treatment. She is in good health, and prior to one year ago, had never experienced excessive worry about any aspect of her life. In this case, we are challenged to understand Ms. B's year-long pattern of excessive worry about her health.

Ms. B is the eldest of three children, born into a middle-class family. Her childhood and adolescence was marked by physical violence in the home. She was a good student and had a steady boyfriend in high school, but was not sexually active. She used a small amount of alcohol and marijuana during high school. She describes herself as "goal-oriented" and "driven." She was apparently able to negotiate the normal developmental challenges of adolescence as well as the challenges particular to her father's behavior with emotional stability. She drank a small amount of alcohol in college, but did not use any drugs. She worked full time while attending college full time, where she met her husband. After graduating, Ms. B married. She and her husband saved enough money to buy their own home. Ms. B has been steadily employed at the same firm, with increasing responsibility, for the past twenty-five years. She and her husband have two teenage children. Over the past twenty-five years she has approached all of her life roles (e.g., adulthood, marriage, home ownership, motherhood) with her characteristic drive and focus.

One year ago, a college friend's cousin was diagnosed and treated for ovarian cancer. After that, Ms. B started to develop worry about her own health, beginning with worry about spine cancer. Once tests came back negative for this, the focus of her worry changed to a series of other cancers: colon, vulvar, brain, and breast. More recently she has been excessively worried about her blood pressure and, now, skin cancer. In addition to worry, Ms. B has experienced a disruption of her sleep, with frequent middle-of-the-night and early morning awakening for one year. She has had a decreased appetite with a 20-pound weight loss over the past year. Although she states that her low libido has not changed significantly since her children were born, she has had no sexual relationship with her husband since the onset of her psychiatric condition. She describes a sad mood and was tearful and sad-appearing. She endorsed a decline in her energy, motivation, and concentration. She views herself as unhealthy. Although she feels like a good person, she is worried about her future and has a diminished self-attitude. However, she is generally hopeful and wishes to live. She has no thoughts of harming herself. She presents seeking relief from persistent health concerns that she views as bothersome and irrational.

Step 5: Consideration of Each Perspective

The Life-Story Perspective

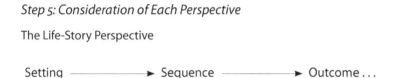

Ms. B's current health worries arose a year ago in the setting of ovarian cancer diagnosed in a cousin of a close friend. Following the friend's cousin's diagnosis, Ms. B first worried that she herself might have spine cancer. After testing allayed her concern about spine cancer, Ms. B began worrying that she had colon cancer, then vulvar cancer, then brain cancer. After her friend's cousin died, Ms. B's worries became mainly focused on her breasts, and she's had multiple mammograms to check out lumps that she's felt on self-exam. Unlike her serial concerns about other forms of cancer, which were each allayed by negative test results, Ms. B's fears about breast cancer have been persistent, despite similarly negative test results. In this case, life-story reasoning could be invoked to help explain the sudden onset of her illness following her friend's cousin's diagnosis and its escalation following her death. And, if her symptoms were less severe and persistent, life-story reasoning could perhaps explain the origin of her illness. However, there are several problems with this line of reasoning. First, there is the possibility that her learning about the illness of a complete stranger was coincidental with the onset of her own illness. In the ordinary course of life, we learn about the illnesses and deaths of others nearly daily. Second, Ms. B's current state represents such a precipitous and radical departure from her usual way of interacting with the world that the life-story perspective seems inadequate to account fully for the origin of Ms. B's psychiatric condition. We conclude that the life-story perspective, while having some explanatory value in her case, is inadequate to explain fully the origin of Ms. B's present illness.

The Dimensional Perspective

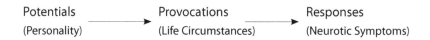

Potentials	Provocations	Responses
(Personality)	(Life Circumstances)	(Neurotic Symptoms)

Throughout her life, Ms. B has always been a very stable and rational woman. She describes herself as "highly organized" and "very goal-driven." Ms. B says that she tries "never to show any weakness," and is generally a warm and cheerful person. At baseline, then, Ms. B is an emotionally stable individual who usually focuses more on the past/future than the present. Thus, Ms. B's temperament rests on the introversion side of the introversion-extraversion dimension, although not on the extreme. Ms. B is not usually preoccupied with her health or any other worries, and has been able to enjoy easy, although not especially close, relationships with her family, friends, and co-workers. She is deliberate and thoughtful in making decisions, seeking to avoid risks. Her temperament may not account for the rather sudden onset of new multiple and persistent health worries (i.e., the initiation of the illness); however, it certainly may explain its features and persistence. Her future orientation, which overlaps with her obsessionality (a discussion of which is beyond the scope of this case book), is affecting her illness-related thoughts and behaviors. She says, "Well, I've always been highly organized and very goal-driven. Sometimes I'll go on a mission, cleaning the house from top to bottom, or, like when we were looking to buy the lake house, researching every single house on the market. My husband says I'm like a dog with a bone. I get hooked on a project and I can't think of anything else until it's done." This same attitude (i.e., pathoplastic effect) shapes how she thinks and behaves in relationship to aches, pains, and freckles,[1-3] consistent with her usual future-oriented attitude and behavior. Although this change represents an extension of Ms. B's usual tendency toward introversion, her current state of excessive concern about her health cannot be explained fully by her temperament. Therefore, we can conclude that although Ms. B's present condition may not be arising solely from who she *is* as a person, its shape and persistence seem in part explained by the dimensional perspective.

The Behavior Perspective

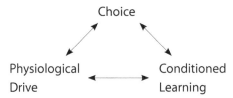

Ms. B is engaging in a pattern of acquired goal-oriented behaviors: seeking medical attention to explain various physical perceptions such as the breast lumps that she detects. Ms. B's repetitive behaviors are something she's doing to reach a certain end and, although they do not appear to explain the initial onset of her problems, they may be relevant to their persistence. In their efforts to pay attention to Ms. B's symptoms, her health care providers have responded to her concerns by ordering diagnostic tests. Although this medical attention has had the cumulative effect of maintaining her help-seeking behavior, it has not worsened the behavior as it does for some patients. These latter patients may visit one provider after another for the same complaint or read one Internet article after another for the same complaint. And even though all of the health care providers or articles agree in general, these patients notice not the agreement, but the fact that the providers or articles didn't give *exactly* the same information.[4] Ms. B is not seeking out the sick role in order to solve another problem, but is visiting providers to relieve a dysphoric state ("that gnawing feeling that things aren't okay, that I'm not safe, came back"). Therefore, for Ms. B, the conceptual triad of *choice*, physiological or acquired *drive*, and conditioned *learning* is less relevant to understanding aspects of her present illness than is her temperament.

The Disease Perspective

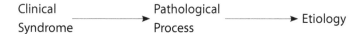

Clinical Syndrome ——————→ Pathological Process ——————→ Etiology

In this case, Ms. B's excessive concern about her health occurs in the context of the clinical syndrome (a cluster of symptoms that frequently occur together) of major depressive disorder. Anxiety, rather than sadness, is the more prominent dysphoric mood (much like excitement or irritability, rather than euphoria, may sometimes occur with mania). Ms. B's present illness occurs against the background of possible depressive episodes in adolescence. Her present condition developed out of the blue (as we doubt the news of a stranger's illness as an important etiologic factor, as opposed to a determinant of the content of Ms. B's worries and doubts). Specific elements of the syndrome of major depressive disorder seen in Ms. B include sleep disturbances, decreased appetite and weight loss, low libido, sad mood, diminished energy and motivation, concentration problems, and an overall view of herself as unhealthy.

Even though Ms. B's medically unexplained complaints are what led to the psychiatric referral, what the systematic assessment reveals is an individual whose major depressive disorder is expressed, in part, by worries about her health. Other depressed patients may present with worries about finances, self-worth, or other things, Ms. B's worries about her health are shaped by the future-oriented and obsessional aspects of her personality.

Hypochondriasis, a cluster of medically unexplained somatic complaints without a syndromic nature and lacking any clinicopathological correlation to disrupted brain function or structure, cannot be well understood from the disease perspective. However, worries about medically unexplained somatic complaints can be understood, in some cases, as manifestations of what we presume to be diseases (e.g., hypochondriacal delusions in major depressive disorder, delusional parasitosis) or of other psychiatric conditions whose status is less clear (e.g., body dysmorphic disorder). A psychiatric condition best explained by the disease perspective is one in which an abnormality in brain structure or function, or a "broken part," causes a particular cluster of symptoms that run a predictable course. Therefore, based on our current knowledge state, disease reasoning sheds much light on Ms. B's excessive worries about her health. Ms. B's hypochondriasis cannot be fully understood as a disease, something she *has,* but she has accompanying symptoms of insomnia, poor appetite, sad mood, and low energy, which represent a coherent cluster of symptoms that run a course together (i.e., the clinical *syndrome* of depression) which is likely to be traced eventually to a *pathology* in brain structure or function, or a "broken part," and *etiology.*

Steps 6 and 7: Formulation and Treatment Plan

Ms. B's internist, neurologist, and gyn nurse practitioner naturally focus on her somatic complaints, for which no medical explanation could be found, prompting her referral to the psychiatrist. Rather than concentrating on just the medically unexplained complaints, the psychiatrist, in contrast, conducts a comprehensive history and MSE, and then considers her presentation from all four perspectives. Applying this approach, two major ingredients shine through: her future-oriented, obsessional temperament and the syndrome of major depressive disorder. Ms. B's temperament can be seen in her thoughts and behaviors. She wonders how she can determine that she doesn't have cancer, which leads her to visit a health care provider who is able to reassure her. For example, Ms. B says, "When the appointment finally came I got some relief. She examined me from head to toe and did another MRI, and this one was totally normal. . . . I could finally relax, and for a little while I was almost back to my old self." Her help-seeking behavior is reinforced by these doctor visits where she gets reassurance. But it is her inability to disprove a negative—wondering how she can know that a somatic symptom does not represent cancer—that initiates the visits and is the main event, which is a problem of doubt. This doubt is part of how she approaches the world—as highly organized and very goal-driven. Thus, the help-seeking behavior is ultimately an expression of who she *is* as a person, which shapes the expression of the major depressive disorder, a syndrome that has come upon her suddenly.

Understanding Ms. B's illness primarily from these two perspectives, dimensional and disease, as arising from who she *is* and what she *has,* provides insight into the primary treatment goals for Ms. B. Although the pathologic etiology and mechanism of the disease of major depressive disorder is as of yet unknown, medication combined with individual psychotherapy is the recommended treatment. Because Ms. B's major depressive disorder has been prominently shaped by her temperament, a primary psychotherapeutic goal would be to guide the patient to respond differently to her somatic complaints. Although there is little evidence to suggest that Ms. B's presentation is arising from something she's encountered or is doing, her illness is occurring, as all illnesses do, in the context of her life. So, another, secondary, goal of psychotherapy would be to combat any demoralization regarding the psychological nature and origin of her current illness ("I know it sounds crazy, and maybe it is") by helping her find an alternative and more adaptive way of understanding her illness. A secondary goal would be to help her interrupt the habitual cycle of seeking reassurance for all somatic complaints.

Case Conclusion

Dr. Hudson recommends a combination of medication and psychotherapy treatment to which Ms. B agrees. Due to Ms. B's adverse reaction to a low dose of sertraline (25 mg daily), he first prescribes the very low dose of citalopram (2.5 mg daily) and then fluoxetine elixir (1 mg daily). However she becomes dizzy and nauseated on each of these medications, and so ultimately is prescribed buproprion, beginning at doses of 50 mg daily and slowly increasing to 150 mg daily, which she tolerates well. In addition, Ms. B is successfully engaged in a course of individual cognitive behavior psychotherapy. Dr. Hudson advises Ms. B to draw on her personality strengths of superior intellect, determination, and stoicism to combat her anxious feelings and maladaptive thoughts/behaviors. She reads extensively about her condition. Each morning she spends at least 30 minutes in cardiovascular exercise followed by another 30 minutes of meditative/relaxation practice. She counters automatic thoughts by writing in a journal throughout the day. After a year of combined medication and psychotherapy treatment, Ms. B feels close to baseline. Despite numerous life events, such as her husband's hospitalization with a life-threatening illness and a co-worker's diagnosis with breast cancer, she experiences no re-emergence of her symptoms. Ms. B continues to take

150 mg bupropion daily and is seen in supportive psychotherapy twice a year.

Summary Points

1 It is important to include a review of systems as part of every psychiatric evaluation, especially for patients presenting with medically unexplained somatic complaints

2 Understanding an illness marked by medically unexplained somatic complaints requires not only a comprehensive psychiatric history and MSE, but also a broad and critical synthesis of the four perspectives

3 Hypochondriacal symptoms can occur as a manifestation of diseases such as major depressive disorder

A Young Woman's Fear of Fat

An Aberration in Feeding Behavior

D r. Berridge meets Ms. A, a 28-year-old woman who had relocated from New York three months prior to attend graduate school. Ms. A is seeking ongoing outpatient psychiatric treatment.

(Dr. Berridge's comments are printed in *italics*.)

Good morning, Ms. A. It's nice to meet you. I received your records and spoke with your psychiatrist, Dr. L, in New York, but was wondering if I could ask you a few questions myself to get to know you better and understand how I might be able to help you at this time.

Sure. That's why I'm here.

Great. Could you tell me a little bit about your parents?

Well, Mom was born in Madrid and lived there until she was 14, when she came here to go to boarding school. She's 51 now and has yet to work a day in her life.

She was a stay-at-home mom?

More like a stay-at-home drunk.

Does she have any other psychiatric conditions besides her alcoholism?

Oh, yeah. She has bipolar disorder and takes lithium. But she didn't gain weight on it like I did. She's naturally thin, for some reason. She's been hospitalized a few times, too.

What about your father—does he drink?

Not at all. He's a professor at Smith. I don't know how he's put up with her all these years. He doesn't have any problems, other than her.

Do you have any brothers or sisters?

Just one sister who's two years older than me. I'd say she's the most "mentally stable" (patient makes air quotes sign) of all of us.

What does she do?

She's married, kids, big Victorian house in Amherst.

Do you see much of her?

Not if I can help it. It's not that she's a bad person or anything; we're just very different. She doesn't work either, except for volunteering at the kids' school. She goes to Martha's Vineyard every summer and—ugh—weighs about 300 pounds.

Is she happy?

Yes, but I can't imagine why. I'd shoot myself if that was my life.

Has anyone in your family ever attempted suicide?

Mom has . . . a few times.

I'm sorry to hear that. How was that for you?

I don't know; I guess I got used to it. She'd get drunk, OD on pills, go to the hospital; that was just business as usual for us. We had a nanny, even though Mom didn't work, so it's not like we missed her or anything.

(Ms. A denies any problems during gestation, infancy, or childhood.)

How far did you go in school?

I'm actually still going. I'm working on my doctorate in human resources now. I've always done really well in school. I majored in economics in college at Hamilton—that's near Syracuse—and then worked as an investment banker in New York for years, but I hated it. I just decided I needed to do something entirely different. So, here I am.

Are you dating anyone currently?

No. I haven't done that for a few years.

What have your relationships been like in the past?

I haven't had that many. I had my first boyfriend in college, when I did a semester abroad in Italy my senior year. Then, about a year ago, I hooked up with this guy I'd known since freshman year, but that didn't last very long either. He's too much of a f——-up.

Can you find another, less offensive way of describing him?

Oh, I get it. Sorry. Yeah, he was a slacker and a drunk.

Thanks. Have you ever used alcohol?

Yeah. I drank some in college, and I guess I'd say now I'm a social drinker—like a glass of red wine when I go out to dinner or at a party. It's never really been a problem. There was one time, a few years ago, when I was working at the investment firm, when I came to work shit-faced. I was just really stressed out and wanted to try something different. It didn't really help though, so I never did it again.

Have you ever had times when you drank so much you couldn't remember the next day what you had been doing?

No, nothing like that. I really don't like being out of control like that. Plus, I don't want the calories.

Have you ever used any illicit drugs?

No, never.

Dr. L said you're a pretty serious person. I think he used the word "perfectionistic." Is that how you see yourself?

Well, I don't do a half-assed job, like some other people, if that's what he means. I've always been like that. I guess I have high standards. But, I'm not all work; I like to play hard, too. I've always liked tennis. It makes me kind of mad that he said that; "perfectionistic" sounds kind of harsh to me.

Would conscientious be a better word?

Yeah, that sounds better. It's not a bad thing, you know.

You're right. It can be a very good trait to have, in certain circumstances, and in moderation. Ms. A, when was the first time you saw a psychiatrist or sought counseling?

In my sophomore year. I was freaking out my roommate, so the RA sent me over to the counseling center.

What freaked her out?

I had gained weight my freshman year—you know, the freshman fifteen—so I'd started skipping meals and exercising, and I guess they thought I had a problem.

You didn't have any issues with eating before starting college?

No, none. I did a lot of sports in high school—I ran cross country and played tennis and soccer. I could eat whatever I wanted, no problem.

What was high school like for you?

It was great. I really liked school. I had friends. I guess I did put a little too much pressure on myself sometimes, but I had nearly straight

As and was on the varsity tennis team from freshmen year on. And I got into Hamilton, which was my first choice, so it all paid off.

Did you ever notice feeling especially down during high school, with all of that pressure?

No, for the most part I considered myself pretty happy.

How was it for you to go away to college?

I decided I wanted to focus on academics, so I didn't go to a school for tennis, and I pretty much stopped playing. And, then, I was a little stressed out with school and started eating a lot of junk food. When I realized how much weight I'd gained, I freaked out. My sister had gained, like, 40 pounds during her first semester, and I saw how Mother reacted to that—all sorts of back-handed comments, bribing her with shopping sprees. When I went home at Thanksgiving, the bitch tried to start in on me too, but I just tuned her out.

How was your mood during that first year?

Pretty normal. Without the sports, it wasn't as easy for me to make as many friends. I mean I didn't have teammates to hang with. But I went out on the weekends, probably not as much as other people. I probably studied harder than most of my friends. I was really into getting good grades.

So, you gained weight and then you started to diet?

I developed a plan for myself where I decided to fast for two days and then eat whatever I wanted for a day. On the eating days, I'd stuff my face with a lot of cereal and candy from the vending machines—a bunch of junk.

And you started exercising?

Yeah, but that wasn't until sophomore year. At first it was just to be healthy, like running three miles a day. That wasn't much compared to how much I ran in high school. Then one day sophomore year I ate like ten candy bars and decided to make myself throw up.

How often did you do that?

Just that once. I felt really bad about it. Around that time was when the RA made me go see a counselor, which was a total joke. That assho . . . that jerk told me I'd been sexually abused, so I never went back after the first appointment.

Had you been?

No!

So you didn't really get help?

No. But, I never threw up again—well, not while I was at school anyway. Then, the summer after sophomore year, I upped my mileage to six a day and tried to eat about 600 to 800 calories a day.

And you lost weight?

Oh, yeah. By February of junior year I was down to 113 pounds.

That was less than before you started college?

Yeah. I was 120 pounds when I started freshman year.

And how tall are you?

5 foot 7.

So sophomore year you were restricting your calories and exercising a lot. You never vomited again, but were you still bingeing?

Only on the weekends.

Did you ever use laxatives or diuretics or diet pills?

No.

Were your grades ever affected?

No. I managed to pull As even when I was starving. Maybe if I'd gone to an Ivy League school it would have been a problem, but Hamilton wasn't that hard.

Were you happy with your weight at 113, or did you think you needed to lose more?

At first I thought I'd look better if I lost more. Then one day I saw my arm in the mirror and got freaked out by how small it was. I also read an article about anorexia around that time and felt like it was describing me. That was after seeing that lame counselor.

Did you seek help again at that time?

No, but I decided to exercise less and eat a little more. My weight was up to 120 to 125 when I left for Italy.

That's impressive that you were able to do that on your own.

Yeah, but losing weight made me feel so great.

Did your period ever stop?

It did in high school for about two years, when I was playing sports, but not since then. It's been totally regular.

(Ms. A is asked about and denies any medical conditions, surgeries, and drug allergies.)

How was your social life in college after freshman year?

Well, like I said, I was having problems getting to know people. Mom thought it would be a good idea for me to join a sorority so I could meet people. So I did, but I hated it, of course. Most of them were just into drinking and having sex. I ended up finding a couple of people I liked, though, but mostly I kept to myself.

Do you keep in touch with any of them now?

Not really.

You mentioned having a boyfriend in college?

Yeah, Carlos. He was hot! He was the first guy I ever hooked up with. But it only lasted that semester. He was Italian and neither of us wanted to keep up a long-distance relationship.

And it sounded like you said you have never been sexually abused?

Right, I never was. (Ms. A rolls her eyes.)

So, when you were in Italy and had a boyfriend, what were your eating and exercise habits?

Well, I had totally stopped running before I went. There were some cool places to hike there, and we did that a lot. I didn't do it to lose weight; I just liked it. I was trying to eat healthy there, but the food is so incredible and I love gelato, so I did end up bingeing on that a few times. But to make up for it, I wouldn't eat.

Did you weigh yourself while there?

No. I didn't have a scale, and it's not like I know what I should be in kilograms.

So when did you come back to school?

That winter of my senior year. That's when I knew I had really gained the weight back, so I started dieting again. After I got back, I started working as an intern for an investment banking firm. I was 22 then. It was a real pressure cooker. I started to binge a lot to deal with the stress. Then I tried purging again, which wasn't so bad this time. I also noticed a lot of mood swings, and that's when I started seeing Dr. L. He tried me on all kinds of meds. I took, like, a dozen different medications in six years.

That's what he said. Looks like you took fluoxetine, sertraline, paroxetine, citalopram, venlafaxine, lithium, valproate, risperidone, and clonazepam. Do you remember all of these?

Yeah . . . Well, some of them.

Did any of the medications work?

I don't think so. And they all made me gain weight, so even if they did, I didn't want to keep taking them.

When you said you had mood swings, what did you mean?

I would just get really depressed sometimes. Like I was really tired all the time and I felt really bad about myself. That could go on for months. Then I'd be back to normal.

Did you notice any changes in your sleep or appetite during these times?

I couldn't sleep as much, that's for sure. I'd fall asleep by 11, no problem, but I kept waking up at 2 or 3 in the morning. Then I'd have to get up for work at 5, so I never could get back to sleep after I woke up. I didn't notice anything different about my appetite, though.

You had to get up for work at 5?

Well, I went to the gym before work every day. It opened at 5:30 and I'd be there when it opened. I'd usually spend about an hour on the elliptical and then do another half-hour of weights every day. Once a week I'd run on the treadmill, just to mix it up. Once there was a fire drill and I wouldn't leave. I mean, they practically had to pull me off the machine.

Was there anything you enjoyed during those times?

Working out and losing weight. That's about it.

And did you ever have really good moods, where you felt way better than normal?

More than a few times, I guess, but they never lasted long; maybe a few days at most. I remember once when I stayed up all night painting my apartment. I was living with roommates then—it was my last semester—and they thought that was pretty nutty. I mean, it was pretty bizarre.

Did you always seem to need less sleep than usual during those times or have more energy?

I definitely had more energy and needed less sleep. I would have so much pent-up energy that I would go out for these midnight runs. I could run for like ten miles.

How about making a lot of plans or starting a lot of projects?

Yeah, I had that. One time I decided that I was going to learn three languages on my own and so I ordered all these expensive language DVDs that I never even looked at. Another time, I decided I was going to write a coming-of-age novel based on my life, and I stayed up for a few days straight working on it. But that didn't really pan out either. When I read it later, it didn't even make much sense.

Did you ever engage in any risky behaviors, or do anything you regretted later?

Well some people thought running in the middle of the night was risky, but, other than that, no.

How long would these times last?

About three days. Maybe four. It only happened once or twice a year back then. Now it happens more. At first, Dr. L thought I had depression, but then I came in all hyped up and that's when he changed my diagnosis to bipolar disorder and started me on lithium.

Was treatment helpful?

Not really. My mood never changed; if anything, it's gotten worse. And with the eating, I would stop exercising and bingeing and restricting for a short time, maybe like a week, but then go right back to it. So it kind of helped a little, but not in the long run.

And you were in treatment for about six years?

Yep. Then two years ago, Dr. L decided I should try a day hospital program, which was the beginning of the end.

It didn't help?

No! Even when I was there I was still going on feeding frenzies. I was also still trying to lose weight when I was discharged. In fact, I felt worse after the day hospital than I had before.

And you've had some inpatient hospitalizations, too, right?

That was about two weeks after leaving the day hospital. I took about twelve over-the-counter sleeping pills. I wasn't trying to kill myself. I was feeling really wound up and I thought they'd help me calm down. I didn't think they'd really do anything bad, but then I got scared, so I went to the emergency room. They thought I was suicidal and so then I went inpatient. While I was there, that first time, my eating got better, but then after discharge I started bingeing and purging and restricting all over again. I didn't go back to work after that, either. I couldn't handle the stress.

Have you intentionally tried to hurt yourself at any time?

No. I was hospitalized the next winter, but I didn't try to do anything. Well, I was cutting my arms then.

Cutting?

Yeah; some of the other girls in the day hospital had told me about that. They said it made them feel less stressed. So, I started trying that then, and it helped.

Sounds like a pretty rough year.

It really was. Luckily I'd made enough money so that I didn't lose my apartment. There's no way I wanted to move back home.

Did things get any better?

Yeah, finally. Last spring he started me on nortriptyline and gabapentin, which seems to have helped a lot. My mood's been really even for the first time I can remember, I'm not cutting any more, and I went thirteen days without losing control with food last summer, which was a record for me. I was able to move here and start school, and so far, so good, at least with the cutting. I still exercise a lot, mostly biking or walking, but I eat enough to make up for it. Like, if I go for a four-hour run, I'll eat an extra 1400 calories.

And the binges now?

It's mainly rocky road ice cream. It'd been down to a gallon once or twice a week. But, with midterms last month, I started back almost every day, and I've been having urges to cut myself again. But I haven't. And I'm not throwing up at all anymore. I've pretty much given that up for good now. When I binge now, I just exercise more. I don't feel like 100% happy. But I'm not feeling sad. I just don't have any real "up" times any more.

And your sleep?

I've been tossing and turning all night.

What about your concentration—how's school going?

It's hard. I'm definitely having a hard time studying, which worries me. So, it seemed like a good idea to get back into treatment.

MSE: Ms. A is a muscularly toned young woman wearing shorts and a tank top. She has biked to the appointment and brings her bicycle into the waiting room. Her gait is assessed as normal. Ms. A is alert and cooperative. She sits quietly, makes good eye contact throughout the interview, with no tremors or tics. She has pale, faint scars criss-crossing her anterior forearms bilaterally. There are no apparent hallucinations. Ms. A answers all questions appropriately, without delay. Her speech is normal in rate, rhythm, and volume and displays appropriate articulation. There is no evidence of thought disorder or aphasia. She describes her mood as "stressed," and her affect appears slightly sad and irritable. She denies any suicidal or homicidal thoughts. She denies any feelings of guilt or self-blame. She is not hopeless, and denies grandiose or persecutory delusions. There are no hallucinations. She has a fear of gaining weight, but denies obsessions, compulsions, and phobias. Ms. A is fully oriented and has a good fund of knowledge with an MMSE score of 30/30. Her intelligence is assessed as above average. Her insight into her psychiatric condition is good and her judgment is good.

The Discussion

Steps 2–4: History, MSE, and Collateral Informants

Ms. A and her psychiatrist describe a ten-year history of disturbed mood and feeding, requiring two psychiatric hospitalizations, plus one partial. Ms. A's mother has bipolar disorder and alcohol dependence, about which Ms. A expresses disdain and bitterness. Ms. A also expresses disgust toward her sister, who is overweight. Ms. A is a hard-working and active woman who is described as "perfectionistic." She expresses strong feelings, especially regarding her mother and sister, with whom she has strained relationships. She has engaged in impulsive behaviors in the past including arriving intoxicated to work, but is generally a dependable and future-oriented individual. She has few, if any, friends and has had only one romantic relationship, which lasted less than six months.

For most of the six months prior to this evaluation, Ms. A's mood symptoms have been well controlled with a combination of nortriptyline and gabapentin treatment. She has not engaged in self-cutting, and has been bingeing less frequently. However, she has continued to engage in excessive exercise and calorie counting to avoid gaining weight.

In the two months prior to the evaluation, just after moving to a new state and beginning graduate school, Ms. A has noticed worsening of her mood, sleep, and concentration. In addition, she has been engaging in more frequent binge eating and has had urges to cut herself. These symptoms prompted her to seek psychiatric care locally. On exam, she appears sad and has diminished vital sense, but an intact self-attitude. She has no psychotic signs or symptoms and her cognition remains intact.

Step 5: Consideration of Each Perspective

The Life-Story Perspective

Setting ⟶ Sequence ⟶ Outcome . . .

Ms. A's current difficulties have occurred in the setting of moving from another state to begin a doctoral program. She has experienced a lower mood, insomnia, impaired concentration, and renewed urges to cut herself. Her binge-eating episodes have increased in frequency. Many of these symptoms and their course are suggestive of a depressive condition, and Ms. A has been taking medication for an atypical form of bipolar disorder. But this mood disorder had been under good control prior to her move, and so the timing of these symptoms may be understood partly as arising from relocation to a new state and starting graduate school. We can empathically understand that she is feeling sad, and perhaps even having trouble sleeping and concentrating, in this new situation. But it is more difficult to understand empathically her desire to cut and binge.

Ms. A also tells a story of growing up in a household with a mother who was alcohol-dependent, naturally thin, and excessively critical of the obesity of Ms. A's sister. She describes her father as high-achieving. Ms. A is disdainful when talking about her mother and sister and clearly holds her father in higher esteem. Life-story reasoning can help explain the timing of the onset of these more-recent symptoms and perhaps the form of the behaviors (binge-eating and urges to cut), but it seems inadequate to account fully for Ms. A's prior psychiatric history and current presentation.

The Dimensional Perspective

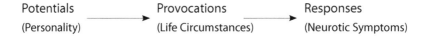

| Potentials | Provocations | Responses |
| (Personality) | (Life Circumstances) | (Neurotic Symptoms) |

Throughout her life Ms. A has been a smart and savvy individual. She is hard-working and hard-playing with strong feelings toward her family members, boyfriends, and her previous psychiatrist. In response to these strong feelings, Ms. A describes engaging in the past in impulsive actions such as arriving at work intoxicated, cutting herself, or bingeing. In addition, she has been unable to maintain any long relationships, all of which suggests her temperament most likely rests on the instability extreme of the instability–great stability dimension.

In addition to this reactivity, Ms. A's underlying temperament is quite perfectionistic. She has very "high standards" and is prone to criticizing herself and others. She focuses much more on the past/future than the present and rests, therefore, on the extreme introverted side of the introversion-extraversion dimension.

Her extreme tendency in both temperament dimensions (instability and introversion) explains many aspects of her current presentation, such as the emotional reactivity to a new living and school environment and the renewed urge to cut. Ms. A describes this as a change from how she had been feeling for the prior six months; but it is, in fact, similar to her usual attitude and behavior, and thus could be explained in large part by her temperament alone. However it is important to remember that individuals who rest on dimensional extremes are not immune to behavioral disorders and disease syndromes. In this case, the dimensional perspective explains many, but not all, aspects of Ms. A's presentation.

The dimensional perspective may not account for the specific form of her attitudes and behaviors (binge-eating and urges to cut) and the course of a cluster of symptoms (acute onset of worsened sleep, mood, and concentration). Although we conclude that Ms. A's present condition may be arising in large part from who she *is* as a person and can be understood partly by the dimensional perspective, the savvy clinician will want to continue to examine the case from the remaining perspectives.

The Behavior Perspective

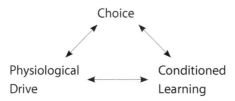

In Ms. A's case, she is engaging (or thinking about engaging) in several behaviors—self-cutting, calorie-counting, over-exercising, restricting food intake, and binge-eating—that are allowing her to achieve certain ends (i.e., they are goal-oriented): to diminish anxiety or to stay thin. The latter behaviors—revolving around a "morbid fear of fatness,"[1] which McHugh and Slavney have characterized as the "overvalued idea" that "one cannot be too thin"[2]—dominate her life, to the detriment of work, school, friends, and health. This fear drives many of Ms. A's activities and replaces all of her other nonwork/school interests, such as dating, socializing, and non-athletic hobbies, thus narrowing her behavioral repertoire.

Anorexia nervosa and bulimia involve goal-directed behaviors and need to be treated as such. However, these behavioral disorders are more likely to occur in patients of certain extreme temperaments and/or in patients who have mood and anxiety disorders. Just as extreme instability can drive abnormal cutting and eating behaviors and extreme introversion can enable some behaviors, like self-starvation, to be sustained, untreated mood and anxiety disorders can also drive and sustain such abnormal cutting and eating behaviors. Thus, Ms. A will also need to be assessed for co-occurring psychiatric diseases as part of the systematic psychiatric evaluation.

The Disease Perspective

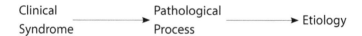

In this case, Ms. A's current illness clearly has the form of a mood disorder (acute onset of worsened sleep, mood, and concentration), most likely bipolar depressive disorder, given the presence of episodes marked by euphoria and/or decreased need for sleep (e.g., staying up all night painting, buying language CDs, writing a novel, going on midnight runs). She had multiple trials of various psychiatric medications, including mood stabilizers, but eventually responded to nortriptyline and gabapentin. Since abnormal moods can drive behaviors, as expected, as Ms. A's mood got better, the cutting and eating behaviors also improved, as did her overall functioning. With either major depressive disorder or bipolar disorder, as with many other psychiatric conditions for which disease reasoning may be appropriate, we have only hints of clinicopathological correlations and etiology. But, based on what we know to date, disease reasoning seems appropriate to explain, at least partially, Ms. A's illness. Thus, given her family history of mood disorder and remission of some symptoms and functional improvement with recent pharmacologic treatment, some aspects of Ms. A's presentation may be explained by a "broken part," an abnormality in the structure or function of her brain.

Steps 6 and 7: Formulation and Treatment Plan

Ms. A's case is complex. She reports a childhood marked by her mother's alcohol dependence and critical remarks about her sister's obesity without apparent intervention by her father, whom she holds in high regard. She is a high-achieving, critical, rigid, and perfectionistic individual who is extremely future-oriented, but who can act impulsively at times. She is intensely reactive, has no close friends, and responds to her feelings by cutting her arms with the false hope of allaying dysphoric feelings, including her fear of being fat. Ms. A has responded to this fear by counting calories, over-exercising, restricting food intake, and—in the past—purging (vomiting) in response to binge-eating. These behaviors are reinforced by short-lived reduction in anxiety and a sense of control.

On exam, Ms. A displays a variety of psychiatric signs and describes a number of symptoms. Her speech is normal in form, but peppered with obscenities and, at times, laced with a harsh and disparaging tone. Her mood seems sad and hostile; she describes a long history of low mood and accompanying changes in sleep, concentration, and self-cutting. After applying the *Perspectives* approach, we can conclude that aspects of her current condition (sad mood, insomnia, impaired concentration) may be at least partly understood as something she *has*, in addition to also arising from something she has *encountered*, who she *is*, or what she is *doing*.

Ms. A may be experiencing a mild recurrence of bipolar depressive disorder, for which a combination of pharmacologic treatment and individual psychotherapy is typically helpful. However, this perspective only begins to explain her presentation fully. If we had not taken a systematic approach, and instead checked her symptoms against the *DSM* criteria for bipolar depressive disorder, we could easily have started and stopped with the disease perspective. In this case, we employed the *Perspectives* approach to reach a fuller formulation and treatment plan. The form of Ms. A's presentation can also be explained partly as arising from who she *is* as a person (the dimensional perspective) and what she's *en-*

countered in her life (the life-story perspective). However, the perspective that best explains the nature and origin of her presentation is the behavior perspective.

In the face of Ms. A's fear of fat, her innately driven feeding behaviors have become deranged via learned conditioning. Ms. A, like many patients who come to treatment seeking relief from the burdens of their abnormal behaviors, has been able to modify and even give up certain behaviors, but has not been able to give up all of them. Although Ms. A has not engaged in self-cutting and has been bingeing less frequently, she has continued to engage in excessive exercise and calorie counting to avoid gaining weight, despite treatment. She rationalizes these abnormal behaviors as she continues to cling to them.

A goal of treatment will be to win her trust so that she is willing to limit her exercise and stop counting calories. While addressing the mood symptoms for which Ms. A now presents for treatment, Dr. Berridge is able to persuade her that changing the exercise and calorie-counting behaviors is necessary to achieve a full recovery. We include Ms. A's case here to offer up a complex case for formulation and to illustrate how the formulation informs a personalized and complete set of treatment recommendations.

Because Ms. A's presentation can be understood as arising from all four perspectives, her treatment plan will encompass all four associated goals. However, we will need to prioritize these goals for her. Although she has relatively mild depressive and eating symptoms, these need to be addressed first so that she will have the ability to work in psychotherapy on her other problems, which have their origin in her temperament and life story.

Although Ms. A's depressive symptoms are not currently the most prominent aspect of her presentation, they are important to address early in her treatment. Given the limits of knowledge regarding the etiology and pathophysiologic mechanisms of most psychiatric diseases, we can't yet speak of a cure for psychiatric disease in the same way we can for other medical diseases. However, we can say that pharmacologic treatments exist for mood disorders. These can at times approximate a cure, especially when coupled with individual psychotherapy. Thus pharmaco- and directive psychotherapy (focused first on persuading her to take responsibility for interrupting all abnormal behaviors and then on providing guidance regarding her emotional instability and introversion) is indicated to address this aspect of Ms. A's presentation. With this combination, we hope that Ms. A will achieve improved mood, sleep, and concentration and thus be "cured" of this episode of major depressive disorder.

A second, and equally important, goal of treatment for Ms. A will be to continue to interrupt and/or stop the abnormal cutting and feeding behaviors. A combination of individual and group psychotherapy is optimal to achieve this goal. Achieving this goal, which will take time, will enable her to concentrate fully in individual psychotherapy in working on the third and fourth goals. She will need to be guided in psychotherapy to avoid provocations (when possible) and responses to these provocations to which she is prone due to her unstable and introverted temperament. In addition, Ms. A may need to rescript her life story to a more adaptive one in which she views herself less as a victim of her childhood and more as an agent of her own ability to change. If she is in a starved state, even if no longer depressed, she will not be able to engage fully in psychotherapy, which will limit its success. However, we have often found that, once a patient's disease and behavioral disorder are treated, the aspects of presentation related to life story fade in importance to the patient.

Case Conclusion

Ms. A's nortriptyline serum level measures 78 nanograms/milliliter (ng/ml), so Dr. Berridge increases the dose slightly, and a repeat serum level is 123 ng/ml. Dr. Berridge meets weekly with Ms. A for individual cognitive behavioral psychotherapy, which focuses initially on behavioral goals (preventing return of self-cutting, eliminating the binge-eating episodes and calorie counting, eating well-balanced meals, and maintaining a daily one-hour maximum exercise schedule, regardless of food intake). In addition, Dr. Berridge refers her to an eating disorder psychotherapy group, which meets weekly.

With Dr. Berridge's support, Ms. A joins a running club whose members, in addition to going on short runs together weekly, participate in monthly community service. Dr. Berridge begins to focus psychotherapy on guiding Ms. A through various interpersonal challenges at school and at home, including with her family of origin. Dr. Berridge teaches Ms. A relaxation techniques, such as the body scan and breathing exercises, which Ms. A uses throughout the day when she feels stressed by school. Ms. A has had no return of urges to cut or binge and, although she still worries about gaining weight, has been able to limit her exercise and eat healthy meals without counting calories.

Summary Points

1 The goal of treatment depends upon the origin of a patient's psychiatric condition

2 Each perspective has a corresponding treatment goal
   • The goal for a life-story disorder is to rescript
   • The goal for a dimensional disorder is to guide
   • The goal for a behavioral disorder is to interrupt (or "convert") the behavior
   • The goal for a disease is to support and, with medication, cure

3 Treatment goals need to be prioritized for each patient in order to maximize successful outcomes and avoid needless interventions

A Lawyer Who Lies and Cuts

Synthesis of a Complex Case

M r. Joel K, a 32-year-old man, meets Dr. Rowe, to whom he was referred by Dr. W, his internist. Dr. Rowe spoke with Dr. W, with Mr. K's permission, prior to this visit.

(Dr. Rowe's comments are printed in *italics*.)

Good afternoon, Mr. K. I'm Dr. Rowe.

I've been dreaming about suicide.

I'm sorry you're feeling so bad. We'll get back to those feelings, but first I'd like to take some time to get to know more about you as a person and your growing-up years. Let's start with your family. Is your father still alive?

No, thank God. He finally died. I'd thought he'd live forever. He was a physicist for Eastern Star, the utility conglomerate that robs you every month. He wasn't bad though. He was just so boring.

How did he die?

A heart attack finally took him down five years ago. He was 75.

Did he have any psychiatric conditions, or use alcohol or drugs?

Negatory.

And your mother?

She was also ancient when she finally kicked the bucket. It took two kinds of cancer and a heart attack to get her. We're like roaches, I guess.

And when did your mother die?

Two years after the old man.

Did your mother work outside the home?

Mom never worked a day in her life. She went to college to study home economics. That's where she met Mr. Science. She got married, dropped out, had kids.

Did she have any psychiatric treatment or use alcohol or drugs?

My mom tipped the bottle quite a bit—I think she was depressed just looking at us kids. After dinner she'd have a Tom Collins, or two or three, before putting us to bed. That's just how it was.

Do you know if she ever saw a psychiatrist or other therapist?

She did see our family doctor, good ol' Dr. C, when I was in high school. I think she got him to give her some mother's little helpers.

You have any brothers or sisters?

Yes, one of each, but they're a lot older. My mom was in her 40s when she had me. I was the miracle, better known as the mistake.

What are your brother and sister like—growing up and now?

My sister's beautiful. She was loose as a teenager; got away with everything. She was the perfect student—graduated from Carnegie Mellon. She could've done anything with her life but she decided to marry an alcoholic dentist. And now she spends her time polishing faux antique brass doorknobs.

Can you tell me a bit about your brother?

Oh, Danny-boy? Daniel's the finest specimen south Jersey's produced in decades. Big grin, wide eyes. He wasn't that smart, but life's a cakewalk for him.

Where is he now?

I don't know. Probably China, Sri Lanka, Zimbabwe. Our dear military pays him to trot the globe while I'm here in Beantown.

Did anyone in your immediate or extended family have any psychiatric treatment or drug or alcohol problems?

Not besides Mother.

I'd like to hear more about you now, starting with your birth and childhood then moving forward in time. Where were you born and raised?

Born in Leeds, England; raised mostly in Jersey. Dad's company moved us around a lot, and of course he never complained.

Did your mother have any problems during her pregnancy with you? Was she drinking or smoking cigarettes then?

Well, she always smoked like a chimney, but I don't think she drank 'til later.

(Mr. K denies any problems during infancy or childhood.)

How did you do in school?

I did well. As and Bs. Law school was harder, but I also tried a lot less.

How about dating?

Sure—I dated a few girls in college.

Any long-term or especially serious relationships?

Not until I met Julie. Well, I guess there was Barbara, too. That lasted for almost a year . . .

When was this?

At Bard. Barbara and I met senior year and she stuck with me through the hell of applying to law school. We both got jobs at the library right after college, but when I moved to Chicago for school she stayed behind at the library. . . . No ambition. I couldn't stand that.

I see. As for other long-term relationships, there was Julie and . . . ?

Is Julie . . . just Julie . . . and everyone who comes in her baggage I guess. Nobody else.

What do you mean?

Well, Julie's not as perfect as she appears. She's been my heaven and my hell. She's no angel—to put it mildly.

In what way? Can you elaborate?

How much time do you have? You're sweet, Doctor, but I'll take up your whole afternoon if you'll let me.

I do want to hear more about Julie, as she's clearly important to you. Perhaps we can continue with more about your history and then return to her later? If time allows, we'll do it today; if not, there will be time next week.

Take the lead, Doc. I'll try to stay on track.

You're doing a great job. It's helpful for me to have a sense of your life, of who you are, what you've been through, and what matters to you. So thank you. Now, a few more questions: what jobs have you held? You mentioned the library . . .

That was just for one year: after college, before law school. I stayed in New York and worked at the library while I figured out what to do next. I'd worked a few part-time jobs in high school and college, mainly as a waiter, the worst job on earth. Then I went to law school, where I didn't do much of anything. Then stayed on at Chicago for a while teaching eager undergrads with stars and dollar signs shining in their eyes.

You taught courses on law?

History of law, actually—why would anyone study that? Then, Julie and I came here to Boston two years ago. I lecture two nights a week at BU Law and defend the public during the day. Bleeding heart, you know? I probably made more as a waiter but altruism enlarges the soul, right?

Sounds like you enjoy your work.

Sure.

Have you ever been abused physically or sexually?

Just emotionally.

By whom?

The parents first. Now, Julie. It's a long story.

And, we'll get back to that. It sounds important. Have you ever been arrested or spent the night in jail?

No. That's my clients' job.

Are you a religious person?

Are you kidding . . . ? No, I'm not a religious person. Are you?

Let's focus on you. I know there are a lot of questions, but we're getting through them, and you're doing well.

What next?

Do you smoke cigarettes? Drink alcohol?

I smoked in law school. And a bottle of wine will last me a week. Pretty boring.

Have you ever tried marijuana or any other drugs—LSD, cocaine, heroin, Ecstasy?

No, I haven't. Maybe I should . . .

I'm glad you haven't. And I'm glad you don't smoke cigarettes any more.

Of course.

Do you have any medical problems?

Low thyroid. That's it.

What medications do you take?

I have it written down here in my phone; hold on a second . . . Levo-thyroxine, 175 micrograms every morning.

Are you allergic to any medication?

No.

Have you ever had surgery?

Appendix out at 21. That was a treat.

Any other medical conditions or medications?

My therapist in college kept wanting me to see a psychiatrist, to stuff me with antidepressants, but I never played that game.

Why did you see a therapist then?

My RA was worried about me, you know with the cutting . . .

You were cutting yourself?

Yeah. Around 17 I got the bright idea that pain felt good. Experimented with needles, razors, dull knives, cigarettes. . . . You should try it.

Have you ever tried to kill yourself?

Of course. About once a year. I'm not very good at it, huh?

Are those urges to kill yourself out of the blue or is something going on?

Oh, they're not out of the blue. I'm usually trying to get back at someone.

And are you also wanting to die?

Well, I'm still here, so I guess not.

Well, I'm glad you're still here. What's the closest you've come?

To death? Ooh, how dramatic. I drank two bottles of cold medicine once. Threw up in the bed. That was lovely.

How many times have you been hospitalized for injuring yourself or for mental illness?

I spent a month before second year law school in the psych ward. I think I left crazier than when I entered.

Have you been hospitalized any other times?

Nope, that was enough.

What brought you to the hospital that time?

Oh, I'd met Julie I suppose. Couldn't fall in love without plummeting into despair. Is that your experience, Doctor?

You were feeling depressed?

Sure—major depressive disorder. That's what everyone said. Makes it sound nice.

What do you think was going on?

I think I was feeling alive for the first time, and I couldn't handle it. Julie was beautiful and confident and sexy. She just took over my mind. I'd seen her for weeks at the coffee shop near school, and when she flashed that flawless smile, I knew she wanted me. We talked, went back to her apartment, and had breakfast the next day. And then I saw her having a romantic dinner with one of our professors. She said it was good for her career. I should've known then.

Known what?

That she was always looking out for numero uno.

That must have been upsetting.

You're insightful. Yes, it was upsetting. I cut and burned and scratched more than ever. I nearly flunked second term but summer came just in time for the breakdown.

Tell me about that.

Well, I slogged over to the hospital and said I was going to slash my throat if they didn't save me.

And then . . . ?

They saved me. Or, at least, they kept me alive. Can't say I'm particularly grateful for that.

You said they diagnosed you with major depressive disorder?

And thyroid disease. That's when I first took the levothyroxine: there, in the hospital.

And any antidepressant medication?

Oh, right, yeah: sertraline—I think I was on 150 milligrams by the time I left there.

Any other treatments?

If you call painting butterflies and doing deep breathing treatments, then yes. After four weeks of that, I was ready to get out of there. I don't think anything had changed. Just got a break from the real world and picked up a label for my problems.

Did you continue with the medications afterward? Did you follow up with a psychiatrist or other therapist?

No. I never even got the sertraline refilled. I just didn't notice a difference. But I still took the thyroid medicine. My internist refills it for me.

So, to recap, you've been cutting or burning yourself since you were about 17, saw a therapist in college, but didn't take medication at that time. Then you were hospitalized once in law school, after saying you were thinking about cutting your throat. You were there for four weeks, were diagnosed with major depressive disorder and hypothyroidism, and took sertraline while in the hospital, as well as levothyroxine, which you've taken to this day. Is that right?

You got it.

And have you ever had times when your mood, sleep, appetite, sex drive, energy level, or concentration changed for days or weeks, regardless of what was going on around you?

My mood definitely changes, but every day, and sometimes I have trouble sleeping or eating, but there's always some crisis going on.

It sounds like you'd describe yourself as moody. Is that right, or do you feel even-tempered?

I think you've got me right.

And it sounds like you're pretty sensitive?

Well, I'm passionate about what I believe in. I'm willing to take a stand and not be a wishy-washy brown-noser, like some people I know.

Do you feel like a trusting person or are you suspicious?

Trust no one; that's my motto.

Are you a punctual person?

What is this, twenty questions?

Actually, it is a series of questions. I'm trying to get a clearer picture of your personality. Would you describe yourself as punctual?

Actually, that's one thing I am. Dependable.

Do you take a lot of risks?

I've never gone bungee-jumping or sky-diving, if that's what you mean, but I like to live a little bit on the edge.

How so?

I like to play little games with people; keep things exciting. . . . Like, in college, I sometimes made things up for my therapist, to see if I could get away with it.

Like what?

Like I told her I was adopted. I don't know why I enjoyed getting one over on her so much.

Besides in college, have you ever been in therapy?

I wouldn't really call that therapy.

So, no therapy since?

No, I've pretty much avoided it until now. You're the lucky one who gets to deal with me.

Well, again, I'm glad you're here and will do my best to help you. Unless there's something I haven't asked about that you think I should know in terms of your history, we can move on to what's been happening recently.

You're the leader.

When you first came in, you told me you were here for depression. Can you tell me more about that?

I can tell you more than you want to know.

Why don't we start with what "depression" means for you?

It means that life is crap, that I'm stuck, I'm cursed. There's no way out. Even death would be torture. . . . Shall I go on?

Please.

It means I'm in a lose-lose-lose relationship and am too much of a coward to get out. See, there are three of us—what do you think about that, Doctor . . . ? A student of mine, Paul, was going through a rough time and I let him stay with us—that started right after we moved here two years ago—and now Julie's in love with him and I'm SO not.

Are Julie and he in a romantic relationship?

Supposedly we all are. I told you that Julie's bad news and I'm a sucker. Well, Paul moving in highlighted these lovely traits. Julie took Paul under her wing, and before I knew it they were getting up early to make pancakes and meeting after work. What could I do? When Julie suggested he join us in bed, I had no choice. I knew it was either all of us or I was out. No one said that but it was plain. And since then I'm a third wheel—an old, spineless, desperate, battered, un-loved, wheel. It's awful. It's just awful.

It sounds painful.

You have no idea. I wake up in the middle of the night with these two fat lumps of bedcovers next to me, and I just want to vomit. Have you ever felt like that?

It must be very upsetting. How long have you been feeling this way?

Two years. At first I tried taking it in stride. Thought "this won't last long—this is just another game of Julie's I have to tolerate." But the game's gone too far. It's been two frigging years and Paul hasn't left. I just want to shoot myself.

And you have tried to kill yourself in the past, with cold medicine? When was that?

That was after Mother died, so three years ago.

Anything since then?

Of course. It's my m.o. I've carved train tracks three layers deep into my quads. Just waiting to strike gold one day and pop a vein that counts.

Again, I'm still not clear—when you do this, is it with the aim of ending your life?

Not really, but I wouldn't care if it killed me. And it feels good. Like I said, I've been doing it for years. I've thought of buying a pistol and swallowing a bullet in the middle of the night. Would make for a pretty awakening for the two of them, don't you think?

Do you have access to a gun?

No. Maybe you can help me with that.

I'd like to help you stay alive and help you feel better. I'm glad you've come to get help.

Good luck.

Any thoughts of harming anyone else?

No. Just me.

How's your sleep been lately?

I'm usually pretty zonked by the end of the day, so I'm in bed by 11, but—like clockwork—I wake up at 4:30 or 5 and can't get back to sleep.

How long has that been going on?

At least a year.

What about your appetite?

I've lost about 20 pounds, which is good because I'd really gained a lot of weight in Chicago. That's some good eating there. I felt all fat and doughy—like their pizza.

You're not hungry?

No. I have coffee for breakfast, force myself to eat a little something for lunch, and dinner—forget about it—I usually don't eat anything at night.

And your sex drive?

Zip.

What about your energy level?

I'm totally exhausted. That's from not getting enough sleep.

I'd like to be able to speak with Julie to get her perspective on you and what's been going on lately. Would that be okay?

What—don't you trust me?

I trust that you're being honest and reporting things as you see them, but sometimes a low mood can color how you see your past and how you view yourself. It's really essential to the evaluation to get someone else's point of view.

Well, if you put it that way—No.

It doesn't have to be Julie: maybe someone from work?

Let me think about it . . .

Although Mr. K is initially skeptical about Dr. Rowe's need to obtain collateral information, he eventually offers the name and phone number of a colleague at BU (where he teaches part time), with whom Dr. Rowe later speaks.

Hi, Ms. H, thanks for agreeing to speak with me today. I understand you've known Mr. K since he first joined the adjunct faculty.

I was here when Joel first interviewed, so even before then. I can't say that we're really close, but I've gotten to know him better than anyone else on the faculty has. He's been over to our house for dinner, and I've gone out with him and Julie, but not so much lately. He's given me the cold shoulder ever since I didn't support him at a meeting a few weeks ago. I'm surprised he even gave my name to you. But, I'm glad he's seeing someone and I'm happy to help. Joel's a good person, I think, at heart, if you can get past his quills.

He's a bit prickly?

Well, yes. I think he has a hard time getting close to people. But he's incredibly smart and talented. And he's great with his students. Unfortunately, he's alienated a lot of the faculty.

How so?

Well, he's too damn opinionated, which isn't good when you're trying to become a full-time faculty member. I mean he's only been here a couple of years and already has blacklisted half the faculty. All you have to do is say one wrong thing and you're on his list. He sees the whole world as black and white, and you're either with him or against him. He doesn't seem to like many people. I used to consider myself lucky to have escaped his wrath. You don't want to be on his bad side.

What do you mean?

Well, he doesn't suffer fools. He's got a sharp tongue and a quick wit, and I've seen him get really vicious. I've seen him attack—not physically—but lash out at some of the faculty he thinks are morons. I think they're idiots, too, but I keep my mouth shut.

Has he seemed different lately?

Liking or hating people, no. But he hasn't been returning my phone calls since that meeting, when I didn't chime in. We run into each other in the coffee shop and have even shared a cup together since then, but he's been a lot cooler. I feel bad for him; I know he's going through a rough time.

How so?

I'm sure he's told you that Paul's turned into more than just a housemate—that Julie's fallen for him.

Have you noticed any other changes in Joel over the past few months or weeks?

He seems angrier, more negative—if that's possible. He looks unhappy and tired. I think he's living on caffeine. I heard he even cancelled a lecture last week.

At BU?

Yes, and that's really unlike him. It seems like he's just given up; he's not taking as good care of himself—some days it doesn't look like he's bathed or combed his hair even. Not that he's ever been impeccably groomed—unlike Julie—but he used to make an effort . . .

Well, thank you, Ms. H, this has been helpful.

Like I said, I'm glad he's asked for help. I've been worried about him.

MSE: Mr. K is poorly groomed but dressed in a jacket and tie. He is alert and cooperative. Mr. K faces Dr. Rowe directly and makes good eye contact throughout the interview. He moves very little and shows no tics or tremor. There is no evidence of hallucinations. He responds to questions without delay. His speech is normal in rate and amount, but is slightly loud in volume. His speech is laced with sarcasm, but is not circumstantial and there is no evidence of thought disorder or aphasia. He reports his mood as "miserable." His affect appears slightly constricted in range and is often inappropriate to speech content. He denies any homicidal thoughts, but describes chronic passive death wishes. He has chronic thoughts of hurting himself, but denies any desire to die at present. He is critical toward himself, for instance saying he felt "all fat and doughy." He appears somewhat hopeless. He has no grandiose or persecutory delusions. He has no hallucinations, obsessions, compulsions, or phobias. He is fully oriented and has a good fund of information, with an MMSE score of 30/30 (the sentence he wrote was: "How can I live in hell when I don't believe in God?"). His intelligence is assessed to be above average and although his insight into his psychiatric conditions is limited, his insight into the need for treatment is good. His judgment is fair.

The Discussion

Steps 2–4: History, MSE, and Collateral Informants

Dr. Rowe is unable to fully win Mr. K's cooperation for the evaluation process, and so the psychiatric history and MSE have not yet been augmented with collateral information from those who have known Mr. K the longest—his partner and siblings who would be the preferred collateral informants in this case. However, Mr. K does allow Dr. Rowe to consult one of his co-workers, who, although not the ideal source of collateral information, does enable the evaluation to be used as a valid point of reference for understanding and treating Mr. K. As Dr. Rowe works with Mr. K, she hopes to eventually gain enough of Mr. K's trust and cooperation to be allowed to speak with the other informants.

Mr. K perceives his birth as a "mistake" and voices little affection toward his immediate family. He describes few close friendships in high school. Other than his present relationship with Julie and a relationship in college with Barbara, Mr. K acknowledges no other long-term romantic relationships with anyone of either gender. At age 17, Mr. K begins to engage in self-injurious behavior for which he sees a psychotherapist briefly, at the prompting of his residential assistant at college. The goal of Mr. K's self-injurious behavior is rarely to end his life; rather, he says he usually harms himself in order to feel "good." However, Mr. K estimates that about once a year he engages in self-harm with the goal of ending his life. Despite these thoughts and actions, Mr. K has been hospitalized only once (after an overdose, while in law school). Other than seeing a non-physician psychotherapist briefly in college, Mr. K denies any history of outpatient psychiatric treatment.

Mr. K feels successful in his chosen profession, although he experiences interpersonal difficulties with his colleagues at the law school, where he teaches part time. Mr. K sees himself as a moody and sensitive person who trusts "no one." Although he is generally dependable, Mr. K experiences pleasure in lying, which he also describes doing to his college psychotherapist. Mr. K's co-worker describes him as "brilliant," but adds that it's been difficult to develop a close relationship with him. The co-worker calls him "too opinionated" and prone to all-or-nothing thinking: "He sees the whole world as black and white." The co-worker views Mr. K as generally disdainful and intolerant of those with whom he disagrees. Over the past few months, she sees Mr. K as angrier and more negative, unhappy, and tired, and attributes these changes to Julie's interest in their housemate, Paul. Mr. K acknowledges that his relationship with Julie has become complicated by Julie's romantic relationship with Paul. Mr. K describes his mood as chronically sad and irritable, feelings that vary in intensity from moment to moment throughout the day. At times, however, Mr. K experiences intense feelings of sadness and irritability lasting weeks or even months. Mr. K says these periods of severe and sustained dysphoria—typically accompanied by difficulty sleeping and eating—are usually precipitated by an increase in stressors, but adds, "there's always some crisis going on." Mr. K presents now for help with feelings of sadness and thoughts of suicide, which have been fairly sustained but gradually increasing in intensity over the past year.

Step 5: Consideration of Each Perspective

The Life-Story Perspective

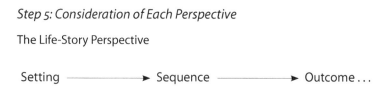

Mr. K's current difficulties have occurred in the setting of a relationship between his partner, Julie, and their housemate, Paul. Julie and Paul's romance has blossomed over the past year, and Mr. K has become a reluctant partner in this triangle. It is in this setting that Mr. K finds himself very despondent and angry, with diminished sleep, appetite, and sex drive; all feelings and behaviors that we can empathically understand given his situation. However, Mr. K is also more fatigued and socially isolated and is thinking more about ending his life, feelings and thoughts that we can less readily understand as arising from his circumstances. In Mr. K's case, life-story reasoning, both recent, which we've focused on here, and more distant, which for brevity's sake we haven't, can help explain some of his present symptoms, but it seems inadequate to account fully for the origin of his psychiatric condition.

The Dimensional Perspective

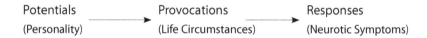

Potentials	Provocations	Responses
(Personality)	(Life Circumstances)	(Neurotic Symptoms)

Throughout his life Mr. K seems to have been a very intelligent, passionate, and volatile man. He has a degree in law, works as a public defender, and teaches part time at Boston University Law School. His co-worker describes Mr. K as "brilliant." Mr. K sees himself as someone who is "willing to take a stand," which his co-worker characterizes as being "opinionated." Mr. K is extremely sarcastic and, at times, rude during the psychiatric evaluation. He reacts strongly and quickly to stressors and agrees that he is "moody." His co-worker says Mr. K's disagreeable attitude and outspoken behavior have alienated him from much of the faculty. But Mr. K sees his opinionated nature positively, regardless of the outcome: "I'm willing to take a stand and not be a wishy-washy brown-noser, like some people I know." He also describes himself as liking "to live a little bit on the edge." "I like to play little games . . . keep things exciting." One of the "games" he mentions playing in the past is lying to his college psychotherapist "to see if [he] could get away with it."

At baseline, then, Mr. K appears to focus more on the present than the past/future and to feel his emotions much more strongly than others. Mr. K's moods are volatile and intense. He is in danger of losing his only long-term partner and perhaps his teaching position, has no real friends, takes pleasure in harming himself, and enjoys the risk involved in lying to others. His temperament clearly rests on the extreme instability and extraverted sides of the instability–great stability and introversion-extraversion dimensions, respectively. Mr. K's apparent lifelong vulnerabilities in temperament may explain some aspects of his current presentation. As discussed previously, it will be important to contact his family to confirm the long-standing nature of these temperament dimensions. However, given the information we currently know, this presentation does not represent a qualitative change from his usual intense self and is one that may be explained in large part by his temperament. In addition, like some individuals who rest on dimensional extremes, Mr. K also reports a history of episodic worsening of his symptoms, and so Mr. K's current presentation may be explained—in part—by one of the other perspectives. Very extraverted and unstable people react quickly and excessively to life-story events and, like those whose temperaments are less extreme, also fall prey to mood disorders, like bipolar or major depressive disorder. For Mr. K, the dimensional perspective may not fully account for the course of the present illness. Therefore, although we suspect that Mr. K's present condition is arising in large part from who he *is* as a person, it will probably be most fully understood when looked at from several perspectives.

The Behavior Perspective

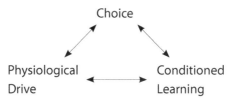

Mr. K states that he is engaging in self-injurious behaviors to achieve a certain end (i.e., his behaviors are goal-oriented: usually cutting to feel better, although about once a year the goal is to end his life; lying to enjoy the thrill of deception). At present, he is experiencing an increase in the desire to end his life, but has not made an attempt. (And, given his history, Mr. K may be lying to Dr. Rowe to achieve satisfaction in getting away with the deception.) Although Mr. K's repetitive behaviors are clearly relevant to his psychiatric history and treatment, they may also be relevant to the origin of Mr. K's current presentation. We will defer further discussion of the relevance of the behavior perspective until later in the chapter.

The Disease Perspective

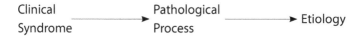

Clinical Syndrome → Pathological Process → Etiology

Mr. K presents with a cluster of symptoms that occur and run a course together (e.g., diminished sleep, appetite, and libido; dysphoric mood; diminished energy and concentration; social withdrawal; suicidal thoughts). Although, at baseline, Mr. K's mood is dysphoric and he has self-injurious thoughts and behaviors, for him these are not usually accompanied by sleep, appetite, and libido changes. Nor does Mr. K usually feel fatigued, withdraw from co-workers, cancel classes, and want to end his life. Mr. K has been treated with the antidepressant sertraline while hospitalized for four weeks during law school. As with all patients, with Mr. K's permission, it will be important to review the record of this hospitalization to clarify his response to treatment. Mr. K's present symptoms cluster and run a course together and hence resemble a syndrome—major depression. Do they respond to treatment for major depression? Mr. K has had only one brief course of psychotherapy—in which he lied to his college therapist—and less than a four-week course of antidepressant medication while hospitalized during law school. Although Mr. K says that the antidepressant (sertraline) did not help, it is imperative to obtain and review the hospital records. If they indicate improvement in his depression in response to the antidepressant, this would support the syndromic nature of Mr. K's current presentation. Based on what we know to date, disease-reasoning may explain some aspects of Mr. K's current presentation (i.e., aspects of his illness may be explained as originating from a "broken part," *an abnormality in the structure or function of the brain*).

If we identify Mr. K's psychiatric condition as the clinical syndrome of major depressive disorder, the next question is can we identify a pathology and/or etiology. In most cases of major depressive disorder, this is not possible. However, in Mr. K's case he is diagnosed with hypothyroidism and treated with levothyroxine. Given his current presentation of the clinical syndrome of major depressive disorder, it will be important to review any recent laboratory examinations of his thyroid function to make sure that hypothyroidism is not the etiology for Mr. K's psychiatric syndrome. Regardless of the etiology, Mr. K's long history of stereotypic major depressive episodes in the absence of treatment suggest a disease of the brain may, in part, explain his current presentation.

Steps 6 and 7: Formulation and Treatment Plan

Mr. K's case provides another excellent example of how applying the *Perspectives* approach can bring clarity to a complex patient presentation. Mr. K's current mood symptoms have come upon him unbidden, as happens with other diseases, and so his current presentation may be understood—at least in part—as something he *has*, rather than arising from something he has *encountered*, who he *is*, or what he is *doing*. However, Mr. K's current presentation may have been precipitated by events in his life story. And Mr. K is an individual who rests on the extremes of two temperament dimensions. In the absence of a systematic and sequential approach, we might attribute all of his symptoms to life circumstances, personality, or mood disorder. Even if we concluded, in the absence of such an approach, that several diagnoses contribute to his presentation, we may well overlook the behavioral aspects of the case and, in doing so, would neglect an important aspect of his formulation and treatment. We have found that applying such a systematic approach to complex cases such as this is necessary to reach a full formulation and comprehensive treatment recommendation.

In Mr. K's case the treatment recommendation is for individual and group psychotherapy—with the goals of rescripting, guiding, and interrupting behaviors—and for pharmacotherapy—with the goal of curing the mood disorder. We include his case here to offer up another complex case for formulation and to provide a springboard for discussing patients whose psychiatric conditions arise from a confluence of sources.

It is well established that borderline personality disorder and mood disorders (specifically bipolar spectrum disorders) frequently co-occur.[1] Treating the mood disorder often mitigates the intensity and speed of the emotional reactivity[2] for these patients (who rest on the extremes of the instability and extraversion dimensions), and is most likely responsible for the better outcomes seen in patients with co-occurring borderline personality and bipolar spectrum disorder. However, as Mr. K demonstrates, more than dimensional vulnerabilities and diseases contribute to the psychiatric condition of these patients. Often they come to us—like Mr. K does—with a life story full of a sequence of distressing events (such as interpersonal conflicts with family and friends, social marginalization, and loneliness) that both result from their temperamental vulnerabilities and contribute to further emotional instability.

Case Conclusion

Within two weeks, Mr. K permits Dr. Rowe to contact Julie, who confirms the history obtained from Mr. K and the co-worker. Mr. K agrees to a trial of nortriptyline, which is titrated to a level of 125 nanograms/milliliter. Within one month, Mr. K's sleep, appetite, libido, energy, concentration, grooming, and social/occupational functioning all improve dramatically. Mr. K's mood improves somewhat, but he still is highly reactive to stressors, which escalate in the months after beginning treatment when Julie and Paul decide to break off from Mr. K and move out of the house and into an apartment together. This event provokes an increase in Mr. K's thoughts of suicide for which a brief psychiatric hospitalization is required. During that hospitalization, Mr. K allows Dr. Rowe to contact his sister, who confirms Mr. K's reports of the family history. Mr. K's sister adds that her brother was a "fussy" baby, a "difficult" toddler, and a "demanding" child. As a teenager, he was extremely quarrelsome and rageful toward their parents. This additional history supports the relevance of the dimensional perspective in the formulation of Mr. K's case. Upon discharge from the hospital, Mr. K actively engages in weekly individual and group psychotherapy to provide guidance on his temperament and to interrupt the pattern of maladaptive behaviors, forged by conditioned learning. After more than a year in psychotherapy, focused on re-training, Mr. K's maladaptive emotional attitudes and behaviors gradually improve. Although his relationship with Julie remains strained, he develops nonromantic friendships with two co-workers, becomes more productive at work, and remains free of self-injurious and other maladaptive behaviors.

Summary Points

1 Every patient presentation should be sequentially examined from all four perspectives so as not to neglect an important aspect of formulation and treatment

2 The *Perspectives* approach is especially helpful in bringing order to the chaotic presentations that often accompany patients who rest at the instability and extraverted dimensional extremes

3 Aspects of the life-story and behavioral perspectives can play an important role in the understanding and treatment of patients with presentations best understood from the dimensional and disease perspectives

A Case of Bereavement

Why Psychotherapy Matters

D r. Gilbert meets Mr. Alfred W, a 30-year-old man who is seeking outpatient psychiatric treatment for anxiety symptoms in the wake of his brother's death in Iraq.

(Dr. Gilbert's comments are printed in *italics*.)

Hello Mr. W, it's nice to meet you. I'm so sorry to hear about your brother.

Thanks.

How are you doing?

Not so good. That's why I'm here.

I'm glad you're here and I hope I can help.

Thanks.

I'd like to start with your family history. Are both your parents living?

Yes. My dad's 66. He retired last year. He worked as an engineer and then a manager in the aerospace industry. He has an MBA. He went to school part time, at night; did that when we were little.

Does he have any medical problems?

High blood pressure and high cholesterol, but he's losing some weight and changing his diet so it's all good.

Has he ever seen a psychiatrist in the past or had any trouble with alcohol or drugs?

No.

And your mother: is she the same age?

She's two years younger—64.

Did she work outside the home when you were growing up?

No, she stayed home with us, but then went back to work as a secretary after we all left home. She's still there.

And how is her health?

She's got high blood pressure, too. She's also been seeing a psychiatrist for about five months, after Tony died.

Was he your only sibling?

There are five of us altogether, but I'm the nearest to him in age. We were always really close.

Where are you in the birth order?

I'm the next to the youngest. My sister Mary is the oldest, she's 40, and next is Sylvia, who's 37. Then was Tony, who was about to turn 33. It was his second tour in Iraq and he was supposed to be coming home for good; he was killed by a roadside IED. That was six months ago. It's been really hard on all of us, especially my parents. It's just so sad; he has three little children. I can't believe he's gone. Sometimes I pick up the phone to call him, and then I remember. It's been tough on my sisters and on my youngest brother, Scott, as well.

Have any of them gone to see a psychiatrist?

Mary was seeing a psychiatrist already because she's had problems with depression. She's the one who talked me into coming in today. This is the first time I've ever seen anyone.

I'm glad you came. I'm sorry it's been so hard, and I will do my best to help you feel better. Was Mary treated with any psychiatric medication?

She's been on an SSRI, I'm not sure which one, though. She says it's helped, along with the therapy. I can't say, myself, because I never knew she was depressed until after Tony died.

Has anyone in your extended family seen a psychiatrist or had any problems with alcohol or drugs?

My grandfather on my father's side had Alzheimer's, but no one else has had any problems.

Any suicides anywhere in the family?

No.

(Mr. W denies any problems during gestation, infancy, or early childhood.)

How did you like school?

I loved it. I was a good student and I got good grades. I was in plays and ran cross country in high school.

And after high school?

I stayed nearby. Wanted to go to a small college; there's a good one that's practically in my parents' backyard. I didn't live with them, though; I wanted to live in the dorms.

What did you study?

Business. I graduated almost ten years ago, now. Since then I've been working as a financial analyst. I enjoy it a lot, and my supervisor is really supportive. They paid for me to get my MBA, too; I got that two years ago.

That's great. Congratulations.

Thanks, it was really pretty easy, though.

Let's go back to college. When you were there, did you drink alcohol?

Sure, I tried it in college, but I never got wasted like some of the guys. I hardly drink at all now, though. I might have a beer or a glass of scotch if I'm at a party. I'm really not a drinker. And I've never used drugs.

Are you currently in a romantic relationship?

No, I'm not real happy about that. I had a girlfriend in college, but we broke up after she moved away for a job. She's a great girl, and we're still friends and everything. I've dated a few other women since we broke up, but nobody lately. I'm not really feeling up to it.

And how many sexual partners have you had in your life, if any?

My ex-girlfriend's been the only one. I'm embarrassed to say we were both virgins when we met.

That's not necessarily a bad thing.

Yeah, but it's pretty rare nowadays.

(Mr. W is asked about and denies any medical conditions, surgeries, current medications, and drug allergies.)

I'd like to get a sense of what your personality is like when you're feeling well. Then, with your permission, I'd also like to talk to your brother or one of your sisters or your parents, too, to get their perspective.

That's fine. Actually, I think my mom is in the waiting room now, if you want me to get her. I was going to take her out to lunch after this.

That would be great, if it's okay with you.

(Mr. W goes to get his mother, Mrs. W.)

Hi, Mrs. W. It's a pleasure to meet you. I'm sorry to hear about your son Tony.

Yes, we're all so broken up by it.

Well, I've been talking with Alfred and wanted to get your perspective on his personality, if I could.

Well, I'll try my best.

Thanks, and Mr. W, please feel free to chime in, too, at any time. Mrs. W, would you describe your son as moody or more even-tempered?

(Mrs. W laughs.) Oh, Al was always such an easy baby and is still always so calm. I don't think I've ever seen Al in a bad mood.

Is he a trusting person?

Oh, yes, but not at all gullible. He's street smart, too.

Punctual?

You bet.

Would you agree with all of this, so far, Mr. W?

I can get in a mood, especially if I'm tired at work, but I guess she hasn't seen that side of me.

Are you a very sensitive person?

Yes.

Mrs. W, would you agree with that?

Yes, but in a good way. I mean, he's always had a big heart. He did have a lot of worries when he went off to junior high; but we took him to the pediatrician and he got over that without much trouble. They were redistricting the schools, and so a lot of his old friends from elementary school went somewhere else for junior high. I think he was just missing his friends.

Did Alfred have a lot of friends growing up?

A fair amount—he was active in sports, running and baseball and such. He always had a few close friends.

Was he more of a leader or a follower? What do you think?

(Mrs. W looks at her son.) I'd say he was more one of the group than a leader. He's just so good-natured; he just got along well with everybody. He was never one to be bossy.

Was Alfred ever someone who took a lot of risks?

Oh, no. The opposite. Al's always been almost overly careful and thinks things through.

And has he ever been particularly self-conscious?

Oh, he can be. I don't think being in front of a crowd comes naturally to him.

Well, thank you, Mrs. W, for coming in and sharing your perspective. Anything else you want to add?

No, just that this has been hard on all of us, but especially Al. He and Tony were close, you know. Alfred's been a great help to us through all of this, though. He's strong; I just hope we're not leaning on him too much. It's really helped me talking to a therapist, so I hope you can help him, too.

Are you taking a psychiatric medication, in addition to the talk therapy?

No. Just talking, and a little anxiety pill to help me sleep, but I don't take that every night. You know, just when I can't stop thinking . . .

Well, thank you again, and I hope you can find a way to heal and make meaning of this tragic loss. Thank you.

(Mrs. W leaves the office.)

Thanks, I'm glad I could meet her. It's really helpful to hear her perspective on you—sounds like you agreed with most of what she said.

Yep.

She said you had some problems with anxiety in junior high?

Yes, but it wasn't about being at a new school or missing my friends, like she said. I mean, maybe that's what set me off, but it wasn't what I was thinking about. I just all of a sudden started worrying about what if something would happen to my parents. I worried about them getting into car accidents or that they would develop a serious illness, like cancer. I couldn't stop worrying about them while at school. So, like she said, they took me to see my doctor. We just talked, but, after a few visits with him, I felt much less worried. I did not have any more problems with anything like that again, until six months ago, when Tony was killed.

Please tell me more about how you have been feeling recently.

Well, everything was going really well. Like I said, I'd been working as an analyst for the last ten years, had my MBA, and had been making my way up the ladder at work. Everything was going great. I'd just bought a new condo, and I'd even been going out on a few dates. I'd hang out with friends from work and I'd see my family most weekends. I missed Tony, but we'd talk on the computer, and he was going to be coming home soon, which we were all looking forward to—especially his wife, Susan. And then the phone call came. I was at Mom and Dad's and we were just sitting down to breakfast, after church, when the phone rang. My dad answered, and I could tell right away that something was wrong. He started crying and calling out Tony's name. He hung up and called Mary who called the others. Everyone came over to Mom and Dad's and at first we couldn't stop crying. But then we kind of just felt raw and numb. There were things to do: we had to plan the service and get ready for everyone who was coming into town for the funeral. I don't remember feeling really anxious until everyone left because I was just so exhausted. A few days after the funeral, though, I started having trouble sleeping.

Sleep problems can vary. Do you have trouble falling asleep, staying asleep, or waking up too early?

I have the most problems falling asleep. I'm really tired, but when I get in bed, I just lie there thinking about my brother and worrying about what it was like when he died. I hope that he wasn't frightened or in pain. I also worry about his children growing up without him. My whole body feels tense, and my heart beats really fast. Sometimes I don't fall asleep until 3 or 4, and I have to get up for work at 5:30. On weekends, I wake up at 4:30 after only a few hours of sleep, which is a big change for me. I've also noticed that my anxiety gets worse during the day. At first I would just feel anxious at bedtime, but now I'm anxious even when I'm at work or even when I'm just hanging out with friends.

Did you try anything to help you feel better?

Yes, I went to see my primary care doctor. He gave me some anti-anxiety medicine to improve my sleep, which helped a bit. I can fall asleep more easily, but I still wake up very early. It hasn't helped with my anxiety during the day, though, at all. Also, there's now times at work when all of a sudden, I feel much more anxious. My heart races, I get sweaty and lightheaded, and my throat feels like it's closing up. I feel like I can't breathe, my chest is tight, like I'm going to go crazy. The first time it happened, I thought I was having a heart attack. I was at work, so I went to the company nurse and had her take my vital signs. They were okay, so I just sat there and waited for the feeling to go away, which took about 10 minutes. It was the most terrible feeling. My friend thought I was having a panic attack. Since then, I've had about five more. Now when I feel one coming on, I go outside. The fresh air seems to help. My supervisor knows what's going on, and she's been really supportive. She helped me to get this appointment with you today.

I have a few more questions about your mood. Sometimes when people have anxiety, they also have problems with appetite or concentration, and sometimes it can be hard to enjoy things you usually like, such as spending time with friends. Have you been having these problems?

No, my appetite has been pretty much the same. I still enjoy socializing and want to do things with friends, I just can't figure out why I am anxious when I am spending time with them. I like being at work because it's busy, which helps my anxiety. I might be a little bit distracted, but no one has mentioned noticing any difference in my work performance.

Sometimes people who have experienced the loss of a loved one might wish they could just go to sleep and never wake up or that they want to be reunited with the person they lost. Sometimes people can feel so bad that they may have thoughts of harming themselves. Have you ever experienced any feelings or thoughts like this?

No, I think a lot about my brother's death, but I never wish I was dead or think about killing myself. I would never do that because I wouldn't want my family to suffer any more.

Not that you should feel this way, but sometimes people feel guilty about being alive when a loved one has died or feel that they are somehow to blame, even though that is not the case. Sometimes they can even feel that they are worthless or flawed in some important way.

Have you experienced those feelings?

No, I know that I had nothing to do with his death and I feel like I'm a good person who is just trying to cope with losing him in the best way I can. I just need some help.

MSE: Mr. W is a well-groomed and neatly dressed, fit young man who makes good eye contact. He exhibits no psychomotor retardation or agitation nor any involuntary movements. Mr. W is tearful at times, and his neck and face flush when he talks about his brother. His speech is normal in rate, rhythm, tone, and volume. It is unpressured and he can easily be interrupted. There is no dysarthria or formal thought disorder. Mr. W describes his mood as "anxious" and his affect is assessed as both sad and anxious. He is attentive during the examination. He denies any passive death wishes or active suicidal ideation, and he has no thoughts of harming others. No hallucinations, delusions, obsessions, compulsions, or phobias are elicited. He describes free-floating anxiety, but no current symptoms of a panic attack. He is alert and able to understand abstract concepts. An MMSE score is 30/30.

Case Discussion

Steps 2–4: History, MSE, and Collateral Informants

Mr. W describes a change in his thoughts, feelings, and behaviors that began shortly after his brother's death and has persisted and worsened over time. His symptoms include both free-floating anxiety as well as anxiety "attacks," characterized as feelings of worry, coupled with palpitations, diaphoresis, and shortness of breath lasting minutes, that occur unprovoked in the evenings (with accompanied trouble falling asleep), at work, and while relaxing at home. When he first experienced these, he was concerned that he was physically ill. With the help of the nurse at his work, he was able to reassure himself regarding his health and never went to an ED for these symptoms. He did see his primary care physician for these symptoms, however, who prescribed alprazolam 0.25 mg bid prn, which he takes on occasion with some relief of anxiety and help with sleep. Mr. W also reports early morning awakening and feeling more distracted at work than usual. He has no wish to die and no thoughts of killing himself. When Dr. Gilbert examines his mental state, Mr. W describes his mood as "anxious" and looks both sad and anxious. Dr. Gilbert's examination confirms a disturbance in Mr. W's affect, encompassing his mood and vital sense, but sparing his self-attitude. Dr. Gilbert identifies no evidence of disturbed level of consciousness, no active suicidality, and no thoughts of harming others. Mr. W has no hallucinations, delusions, obsessions, compulsions, or phobias. Of note, Mr. W has a childhood history of transient anxiety; however, he has always excelled socially, athletically, academically, and occupationally. He is generally a cautious and self-conscious man who, until now, has faced only the typical developmental challenges. He is hoping to find a romantic partner and he has begun to go out on dates. He reports never using any illicit substance and does not regularly smoke cigarettes or drink alcohol.

Step 5: Consideration from Each Perspective

The Life-Story Perspective

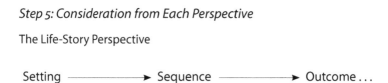

The onset of Mr. W's current difficulties clearly occurred after the sudden death of his brother six months prior. Since that time he's been experiencing not only sadness, but anxiety and bouts of panic. He also has prominent problems with sleep and concentration. This cluster of symptoms can easily be understood in a meaningful way as arising from the loss of his brother. We can empathically understand how he can feel sad, anxious, and distracted, and have trouble sleeping in the face of such an immense personal loss. In this case, life-story reasoning can explain his symptoms and seems adequate to account fully for the origin of Mr. W's psychiatric condition.

The Dimensional Perspective

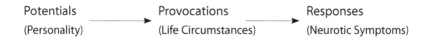

Mr. W has been a sensitive, yet easy-going and even-tempered, person who has been prone to worry, but overall has steered a steady course in life. At baseline, then, Mr. W appears to be focused a bit more on the past/

future than the present and to feel emotions slightly more strongly than others. Thus, he trends toward the introverted and instability side of the introversion-extraversion and instability–great stability dimensions, respectively. However, given the good relationship with his family, friends, and co-workers, we do not see his temperament as resting on the extreme of these dimensions. Mr. W's long-standing tendency toward the introverted and instability side of these aspects of his temperament (confirmed by his mother) may explain some aspects of his current presentation, such as the significant anxiety. However, he and his mother describe this presentation as a marked change from how he usually handles difficulties and one that, even in the face of such a massive loss, surely cannot be explained by his temperament alone. Mr. W presents with psychiatric symptoms that are an extreme form of his usual attitude and behavior. Although helpful in understanding Mr. W's current state, the dimensional perspective cannot account for the timing of the onset of his symptoms, nor the course they have run. The new onset of this particular cluster of phenomena is not accounted for by the logic of dimensional reasoning, which is based in the recognition of enduring characteristics. Therefore, we see Mr. W's present condition as being *shaped* by who he *is* as a person, but not *arising* from who he is as a person. We conclude that Mr. W's presentation, therefore, is not best understood from the dimensional perspective.

The Behavior Perspective

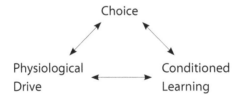

It appears that Mr. W is not engaging in any altered pattern of behaviors, and so the behavior perspective does not seem to be relevant to the origin of his current presentation.

The Disease Perspective

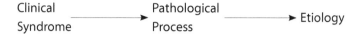

Clinical Syndrome → Pathological Process → Etiology

In this case, one aspect of Mr. W's presentation takes the syndromic form of panic disorder. In panic disorder, as in other psychiatric conditions for which disease-reasoning may be appropriate, we have only hints of clinicopathological correlations and etiology. Nevertheless, based on what we know to date, disease-reasoning might be appropriate to explain part of Mr. W's present condition: the intense feelings of worry, palpitations, diaphoresis, and shortness of breath that come upon him unprovoked in a variety of settings. Other evidence supporting this diagnosis is Mr. W's childhood history of anxiety and panic. Mr. W is clearly heartbroken about the loss of his closest sibling, an aspect of his psychiatric condition less readily explained by a "broken part" of the brain, but one that could provoke the onset of panic disorder. However, loss also provokes "wellings" of grief, an important phenomenon to consider here. But grief and its wellings tend to have a time-limited course, and, in this case, Mr. W's bouts do not have the typical form of welling and are increasing in frequency and intensity, lending further support to the diagnosis of panic disorder in this case.

Even in a patient with panic disorder we can't demonstrate an abnormality that is corrected by medication. However, medications can be helpful in preventing and mitigating the attacks. Mr. W's precipitous onset of symptoms after the death of his brother suggests more than just a disease of the brain as an explanation for his current presentation.

Case Conclusion

We present the case conclusion here to provide a background to the rest of the discussion. Given the diagnosis of panic disorder, Dr. Gilbert recommends a combination of citalopram 20 mg daily to reduce the frequency of panic attacks, combined with individual supportive and cognitive behavioral psychotherapy, which Dr. Gilbert provides. Dr. Gilbert and Mr. W meet weekly for several months and Mr. W's anxiety abates, his sleep and concentration return to normal, and his grief gradually lessens. Mr. W eventually resumes his usual activities, including dating, which continues to be an area of frustration for Mr. W. Dr. Gilbert and Mr. W continue to meet regularly to discuss this and other issues. After three years, Mr. W begins a new romantic relationship and falls in love. Feeling back to his usual mood, the citalopram is stopped. He remains well for about a year, at which time he develops new onset hypercholesterolemia and becomes worried about his health and the future in general. He believes the increased anxiety may have been triggered by his parents' trip to Hawaii and the sudden death of a friend's husband from cardiac arrest. Dr. Gilbert restarts citalopram at 10 mg daily and engages Mr. W in a very brief course of psychotherapy, which focuses on these anxieties. One year later, he is back to his usual self and doing very well. He now sees Dr. Gilbert every six to twelve months for medication monitoring and supportive psychotherapy. Last year, he became engaged, and he is looking forward to his upcoming wedding.

Steps 6 and 7: Formulation and Treatment Plan

Mr. W's case allows us to demonstrate the way a patient presentation is approached sequentially using the perspectives, but his case also shows how the perspectives may be synthesized for a fuller understanding of a patient. Mr. W's presentation can be understood partly as something he *has* and as an outgrowth of his temperament (who he *is*). However, Mr. W's current presentation is most clearly arising from something he has *encountered*. Although there are some who suggest that bereavement is a psychiatric disease, most concur that grief is best thought of as a normal response to loss rather than as a pathological condition.[1, 2] Although an explanation of aspects of Mr. W's case, such as his panic attacks, may benefit from disease-perspective thinking, viewing his presentation only from the disease perspective severely limits a complete understanding of his condition and treatment.

Mr. W describes acute distress following the death of his brother, characterized by a change in mood to sadness and anxiety and with accompanying changes in energy, concentration, sleep, and appetite. On Dr. Gilbert's evaluation he clearly appears bereaved. Although we have applied the *Perspectives* approach and can conclude that Mr. W's current condition is best thought of as arising from a life event, there are elements of his presentation that have their origin in temperament and brain function. By taking such a systematic approach to formulation, we can confidently recommend a specific combination of pharmacologic and psychotherapy treatments.

We include Mr. W's case here not only to offer up a complex case for formulation, but also to illustrate several points. First, this case shows how a thorough history and MSE, which is integral to the *Perspectives* approach, marks the beginning of the psychotherapeutic relationship. Mr. W valued having a professional who took a complete history and asked a lot of questions. Second, this case demonstrates the power of the *Perspectives* approach. It is a method that enables the clinician to understand the fundamental nature and origin of a clinical psychiatric condition. Awareness of a presentation's essential nature and origin then allows the clinician to systematically formulate the case and clearly define treatment goals, which then allows her to thoughtfully select targeted treatment intervention. Appreciating a patient presentation in this way, the clinician can then initiate pharmacotherapy and/or psychotherapy with specific treatment goals in mind. In Mr. W's case, he was started on citalopram to cure his panic disorder. Third, pharmacotherapy is only one aspect of Mr. W's overall treatment; the role of psychotherapy is large. Mr. W appreciated the opportunity to meet with someone regularly who would listen to him; someone he knew would be available in the event of a crisis. Through psychotherapy, Dr. Gilbert helped Mr. W make personal meaning of his tragic loss. She helped Mr. W understand his temperament and guided him through his responses to new and ongoing stressors. And, using cognitive behavior techniques, she helped him deal with panic attacks. Mr. W said that he liked seeing one person for both medication and psychotherapy, as he felt that Dr. Gilbert understood him in a way that could not be conveyed via a third-party psychotherapist.

Summary Points

1 After a sequential consideration of the patient's presentation from each of the four perspectives, it is necessary to synthesize one's findings in order to understand the patient as a whole

2   Psychotherapy begins with the psychiatric evaluation

3   The *Perspectives* approach guides treatment, by pharmacotherapy and/or psychotherapy, depending on the nature and origin of the psychiatric condition

4   The *Perspectives* approach facilitates the targeted use of different psychotherapeutic modalities (an essential part of treatment for patients with all psychiatric conditions) with goals specific to the formulation

· The goal for a life-story disorder is to rescript

· The goal for a dimensional disorder is to guide

· The goal for a behavioral disorder is to interrupt (or "convert") the behavior

· The goal for a disease is to support and, with medication, cure

Summary

I keep six honest serving-men
(They taught me all I knew);
Their names are What and Why and When
And How and Where and Who.
  —from Rudyard Kipling's *The Elephant's Child*
              in *Just So Stories*, 1902

The Perspectives of Psychiatry puts to use psychiatry's unifying concepts by introducing a practical framework for approaching psychiatric evaluation and treatment development. When applied to patients, the *Perspectives* approach builds on the *DSM* and biopsychosocial models to provide a systematic consideration of all facets of an individual's psychiatric presentation, leading to treatment formulation for the whole person. While building on what is done in medicine, the approach goes beyond traditional reasoning about the causes of symptoms, signs, and syndromes to also evaluate other aspects of a patient's condition best *not* construed as resulting from disease. Rather, four distinct natures (perspectives) of psychiatric conditions are considered systematically to see how they illuminate different aspects of what is happening to the patient.

In medically ill patients, clinicians routinely ask: What syndrome does the patient's condition resemble? Why is he or she experiencing this syndrome? This "categorical" perspective implies that the condition results from a broken part in the brain (disease) and explains many but not all psychiatric presentations. The approach articulated here also considers alternative perspectives to explain the patient's condition with questions such as: When in the life story is the problem surfacing? What is the patient doing that might be habitually driving the condition? Who is the individual in whom the problems are occurring? This case book provides a practical approach for incorporating such questions into the evaluation of psychiatrically ill patients so as to better understand and develop treatment for the whole person.

Our use of the *Perspectives* approach over the last two decades has sharpened and clarified our clinical reasoning. It has allowed us to develop a complete range of treatment recommendations tailored to several specific aspects of each person's condition. And it has helped us collaborate effectively with our patients and with other clinicians involved in their care. We hope this case book, with its step-by-step illumination of the *Perspectives* approach, will help all clinicians—especially those new to the field, such as medical students, residents, and junior psychiatrists—formulate cases and treat individuals with psychiatric conditions in a more reasoned and individualized manner, while helping foster collaboration with patients and other clinicians.

Appendix A. The Psychiatric Evaluation

Evaluation Guide

NOTE: *Before starting the interview, state the limits of confidentiality: i.e., comments will be kept confidential except for reports of self-harm, harm to others, and history of or current sexual/child abuse, or in the case of a medical emergency or court order/subpoena.*

Date of Evaluation:	**Time:**
Informants and Patient Contacts	
Identifying Data and Chief Complaint	Emergency Petition? ☐Yes ☐No Voluntary? ☐Yes ☐No
Family History **Father** Age, Health, Education, Occupation, Personality, Relationship	
Mother Age, Health, Education, Occupation, Personality, Relationship	
Siblings (specify biologic relatedness) Age, Health, Education, Occupation, Personality, Relationship	
Extended Family Medical and Psychiatric History Include Neurological or Psychiatric Illness or Hospitalizations, Substance Use Disorders, Attempted or Completed Suicides	
Personal History **Gestation and Birth** **Early Development and Milestones** **Childhood Health** **Social Position** **Home Atmosphere**	

Behavior Symptoms Fires, Fighting (with other children; teachers), Truancy, Animal Cruelty, Enuresis, School Refusal	
Education Age at Entry, Highest Level or Grade Completed, Age at Graduation, Academic Performance, Special Education Requirements	
Occupations Age at Starting Work, Jobs Held, Longest Job, Last Worked, Military Service, Current Income	
Menstrual History Age at Menarche/Menopause, Regularity of Menses, LMP	
Sexual History Age at First Sexual Activity, Number of Partners, Sexual Preference, Contraception and Safe Sexual Practices, Sexual Abuse (reported?)	
Marital History or Other Significant Relationships Duration of Acquaintance, Length of Unions, Age, Health, Education, Occupation, Personality of Spouse(s) and Quality of Relationships	
Children (in chronologic order) Age, Health, Education, Occupation, Personality, and Relationship	
Living Situation Chronology of Living Situations since Childhood	
Religious Affiliation	
Legal History Arrests, Convictions, Total Jail Time, Time Served, Solitary Confinement, Current Parole or Probation	

Substance Use History

Drug	Route	Age at First Use	Current Use and Duration	Maximum Use	Last Use	Longest Abstinence Date/Length/ Context	Withdrawal Symptoms
Tobacco			Pack years				
Ethanol	p.o.						
Marijuana							
Cocaine	Intranasal						
	Smoke						
	IV						
Heroin	Intranasal						
	Smoke						
	IV						
Others Amphetamines, BZD, LSD, MDMA, PCP, Solvents, Caffeine							

Substance Abuse Treatment Episodes:

Past Medical History:

Allergies:

Current Medications (Include OTCs/herbals):

Outpatient Physicians:

Review of Systems

Constitutional	Fever/sweats/chills		Weight loss/gain		Fatigue	
HEENT, Neck	Dysphagia		Vision changes		Hearing loss	
Pulmonary	Dyspnea		Cough		Phlegm/blood	
Cardiovascular	Chest pain		Edema		Claudication	
GI	Nausea Vomiting		Constipation Diarrhea		Hematochezia Melena	
GU	Dysuria Hematuria		Discharge Pain		Bleeding	
Musculoskeletal Dermatologic	Myalgias Rashes Joint pain / swelling					
Neurologic	HA Numbness/tingling Dizziness Lightheadedness Weakness Seizures					
Endocrine	Thyroid disease Diabetes					
Heme/Lymph/ Immune	Easy bruising/bleeding					

Premorbid Personality

Social Relations	To Family: Attachment / Dependence: To Friends: Assertive / Submissive:
Interests	Books: Movies: Music: Other:
Enduring Traits (circle best descriptors)	Optimistic / Pessimistic Suspicious / Trusting Even-tempered / Moody Carefree / Worrier Controlled / Demonstrative Dependent / Independent Cautious / Impulsive Frugal / Generous Leader / Follower Solitary / Sociable Patient / Impatient Strict / Easy-going Confident / Self-doubting Unreliable / Reliable Calm / Anxious Sensitive / Thick-skinned Neat / Messy Self-conscious / Unconcerned about what others think
Standards	Moral Religious
Energy	Sustained output / fitful Initiative Able to complete projects
Fantasy Life Daydreams	Frequency Content
Habits	Eating: Sleeping: Grooming:

Informants for
Personality Assessment:

Past Psychiatric History

Include chronology of psychiatric problems from first onset (including childhood), the associated symptoms including vegetative symptoms, thoughts of suicide or attempts, types of treatments received, including medication trials, and their outcomes.

_____

_____

_____

History of Present Illness

Mental Status Exam

Appearance **General behavior**	Grooming: good / fair / poor Disheveled: yes / no Clothing: own / hospital Eye contact: good / fair / poor Psychomotor agitation or retardation: Abnormal involuntary movements:
Speech form and content **Language** **Associations** **Form of thought**	Speech rate: fast / slow / normal Rhythm: normal or absent Volume: very soft / soft / normal / loud / very loud Tone / Prosody: Pressured: no / yes Can be interrupted: no / yes Dysarthric: yes (slurring yes / no) / no FTD: yes / no Sample of speech:
Mood, Affect **Self-attitude** **Vital sense** **SI/HI/PDW**	Stated mood: Objectively appears: Vital sense (Physical well-being): good / poor Self-attitude: good / poor Hopefulness for the future: Passive death wish: thoughts / intent / plan to harm self: thoughts / intent / plan to harm others:
Abnormal perceptions and illusions	Hallucinations (visual / auditory / olfactory / tactile / gustatory):
Delusions	
Anxiety	Obsessions: Compulsions: Phobias: Panic attacks / Free-floating anxiety:
COGNITION **Intelligence** **Abstraction** **General information**	Level of arousal: Alert Drowsy Somnolent Comatose Abstraction: Estimated IQ: President:
Judgment **Insight**	Situation testing:
Scales, MMSE	Total score: /30 missed items:

Physical Examination

Vital Signs	Wt	BMI	T	HR	RR	BP
HEENT and Neck						
Pulmonary/ Back						
Cardiac/ Vascular						
Abdomen				Abdominal circumference:		

GU/GYN	
Skin/Extremities	
Reflexes	Cranial nerves:
	Motor:
	Sensation:
	Cerebellar:
	Gait:

Data/Labs:

CXR:

EKG:

RBC folate:
B_{12}:
TSH: Mag:
RPR:
Pregnancy (urine/serum) hCG:
Utox:
Serum volatile screen:
UA:
Other:

Formulation

_____
_____
_____
_____
_____
_____
_____
_____
_____
_____
_____

Diagnostic Impression

Axis I	
Axis II	
Axis III	
Axis IV	Acute: Enduring:
Axis V	Current: Past year:

Risk Assessment
Consider Family History of Suicide, Past Attempts by Patient, Lethality, Current Mental State, Past Violent Acts toward Others, Current Thoughts to Harm Others, Unpredictability

Initial Plan
Admission Type, Observation Status, and Initial Treatments, including Medications:

Appendix B. The Mental Status Examination

In chapter 2 we provided the key content of the Mental Status Examination (MSE) (see table 2.1). Table B.1 here presents the same information in a format that can be used at the bedside. Although the MSE has a specific content, and should be administered in a systematic way, many examiners develop their own individualized method of administration. The versions of the MSE presented in this book are meant to serve as ways to "jog" the memory of the examiner when performing the MSE.

Much of what follows is adapted from the book *Psychiatric Aspects of Neurologic Diseases—Practical Approaches to Patient Care,* by Lyketsos et al. (2008). These authors offer a comprehensive and straightforward review of the entire psychiatric examination and this book is strongly recommended to the reader. Only the MSE will be presented here, and the commentary should be viewed as merely a guide.

Table 2.1 offers a quick overview of the parts of the MSE and is borrowed directly from Lyketsos et al. (2008). It highlights the seven main sections of the MSE: (1) appearance/behavior, (2) speech, (3) mood and affect, (4) abnormal perceptions, (5) content of thought, (6) insight and judgment, and (7) cognition. Under each section is a list of the minimum topics to analyze.

Table B.1 presents the same categories for analysis, but provides them in a format that might be more useful for bedside administration. It is meant to be "filled out" with at least the minimal information required for a complete MSE. Minimal information is often not enough, which is why the table contains "Other" areas throughout. Below we will look at each category of the MSE in turn to highlight the importance of gleaning information.

1. *Appearance/Behavior.* This part of the MSE provides the examiner with a chance to record characteristics and develop a "gut instinct" about the patient. Trained physicians use their eyes to examine a patient even before any words are exchanged. What is the patient's physical appearance? Is she fully awake? Drowsy? Does she appear her stated age? Is she well-nourished? Pregnant? Unkempt? What about her body posture? Is she slouching in her chair? Sitting upright? Does she have good eye contact? What about the patient's behavior? Is she behaving in a manner consistent with the context of the assessment? What is her predominant demeanor? Is she crying? Laughing? Angry? Agitated? Restless? Is she cooperative?

2. *Speech*. Although much of an interview involves listening to the content of what a patient says, time must be spent analyzing the speech itself. In many instances, asking the patient to talk about a neutral subject (such as the weather) may help the examiner focus more on speech characteristics. Does the patient have an appropriate range in volume? Is he constantly yelling? Talking softly? What about the rate and rhythm? Is it appropriate? Fast? Slow? Too variable? Is the patient's speech fluid, or does it come in spurts? Does he show signs of latency?

This is the examiner's chance to analyze the patient's pragmatics of talk and to record any evidence of thought disorder or language disorder. Are there signs of circumstantial thought? Echolalia? Flight of ideas? What about evidence of aphasia? Grammatical errors? Errors in meaning? Does the patient seem to understand the questions asked? What about what is asked of him? Can he follow directions?

3. *Mood/Affect*. This section of the MSE has a few more required or essential questions than others. Because answers given here may mark the difference between a hospital admission (suicidal/homicidal ideation) and a release to home, this section has huge implications for the patient. The patient's reported mood should be a direct quote from the patient when asked a question such as "How is your mood right now?" The examiner then assesses the patient's mood and determines if it is congruent with the reported mood. Now, what about the patient's mood itself? Does it fluctuate appropriately (euthymic)? Is it stable? Flat? How is the patient's self-attitude? Her sense of worth? What about her energy level or sense of well-being (vital sense)? Does she find pleasure in what she usually does? Does she not find pleasure in anything (anhedonia)? It is also important to determine if the patient's current mood is similar to her usual mood. If not, can the change be related to recent life events?

4. *Abnormal Perceptions*. A *hallucination* is a perception in the absence of an external stimulus. An *illusion* is a misperception or misinterpretation of a real external stimulus. Some clinicians have difficulty administering this part of the MSE—that is, they have a problem asking questions in a way that elicits valid responses—but, like all other sections, it is vital. Simply asking the patient "Do you have hallucinations? Do you have illusions?" is not enough. Lyketsos et al. (2008) suggest that one way to ease into this section is to talk about hypnagogic (when falling asleep) and hypnopompic (when awakening) experiences. The following question could be used as a lead-in. "When falling asleep or waking up, some people see things or hear things that they can't really explain. Have you ever experienced anything like this?" From there, let the discussion flow to questions like: "Some people see things and hear things that others don't. Have you ever experienced this?" and "Some people are able to notice things in the world that others aren't able to, for example, noticing a snake when others see a rope. Have you ever experienced this?" Collateral information can be helpful in clarifying the history of the patient's experience of these phenomena (but that collateral would be collected via history in addition to direct examination of the patient).

5. *Content of Thought.* A *delusion* is a false belief based on an incorrect inference about external reality. A delusion is a belief/thought whereas *hallucinations* and *illusions* are perceptual experiences and it is important to differentiate. Collateral information about the interviewee's religion and culture and what is considered "normal" is important for this section. The questions that can be asked here are plentiful, but some examples would include: "Some individuals hold beliefs that seem bizarre or unbelievable to others . . . do you?" (delusions); "Do you notice your thoughts tending to focus on anything specific during the day?" (obsessions); "Do you have any rituals you use to get rid of thoughts you have, or to be safe?" (compulsions); "Some people are deathly afraid of heights. Is there anything you are deathly afraid of?" (phobias). Just as it is important to differentiate delusions from hallucinations and illusions, it is important to separately list delusions, obsessions, compulsions, and phobias. They often lend themselves to different diagnoses.

6. *Insight/Judgment.* Lyketsos et al. (2008) explain that *insight* refers to a patient's awareness of his or her circumstances. "Do you think there is something wrong with your health?" "How is your memory? Are you having problems with it?" "Have you been getting along with your family?" Again, collateral informants are instrumental. *Judgment* refers to a person's ability to assess a situation, consider the facts and issues, and draw an appropriate conclusion. It is best to make the questions in this section relevant to the patient. For example, if a patient is about to enter an alcohol rehabilitation program, you could ask: "What would you do if you saw someone in your program drinking alcohol?"

7. *Cognition.* This grand finale of the MSE not only brings together what the examiner has noticed throughout the exam, but it provides the opportunity to formally assess cognition. In too many cases, this section gets condensed down to the performance of the patient on the Mini-Mental State Examination (MMSE). Although the MMSE should be administered, the examiner should feel free, and encouraged, to make additional comments about aspects of the patient's cognition. For example, if the examiner notices that the patient is having difficulty remembering aspects of her recent life, this could be noted under "memory." If the patient consistently loses focus during the exam, note it under "attention." If small talk during administration reveals that the patient does not know the current president's name, note it under "fund of knowledge." Level of consciousness should always be noted in this section.

TABLE B.1 *"Bedside" Mental Status Examination*

1	**Appearance**	Appearance: Grooming: Clothing: Eye contact: OTHER:
	Behavior	Behavior: Demeanor: Cooperative? OTHER:

2	Speech	Volume:
		Rate:
		Rhythm:
		Fluidity:
		Spontaneity:
		Latency:
		Thought disorder?
		Language disorder?
		Question comprehension?
		Ability to follow instructions?
		OTHER:

(continued)

3	**Mood/Affect**	Reported mood:
		Self-attitude:
		Suicidal ideation?
		Plan?
		Assessed mood:
		Vital sense:
		Passive death wish?
		Stability:
		Reactivity:
		Appropriateness:
		Homicidal ideation?
		Plan?
		OTHER:

4	Abnormal Perceptions	Illusions:
		Hallucinations:
		OTHER:
5	Content of Thought	Delusions:
		Obsessions:
		Compulsions:
		Phobias:
		OTHER:

(continued)

6	Insight	Insight: OTHER:
	Judgment	Judgment:
7	Cognition	Level of consciousness: SCALES: MMSE: ____/30 OTHER:
		Orientation: Memory: Praxis: Language: Abstraction: Fund of knowledge:

Cognition (continued)	Attention:	
	Calculation:	
	Executive function:	
	OTHER:	

References

Chapter One: An Introduction

Epigraph. Wallace DF. *This Is Water.* New York: Little, Brown and Company, 2009.

1. Schurman RA, Kramer PD, Mitchell JB. The hidden mental health network: Treatment of mental illness by nonpsychiatrist physicians. *Arch Gen Psychiatry* 42:89–94, 1985.

2. Regier DA, Narrow WE, Rae DS, Manderscheid RW, Locke BZ, Goodwin FK. The de facto US mental and addictive disorders service system: Epidemiologic catchment area prospective 1-year prevalence rates of disorders and services. *Arch Gen Psychiatry* 50:85–94, 1993.

3. Engel GL. The clinical application of the biopsychosocial model. *Am J Psychiatry* 13:535–544, 1980.

4. McHugh PR, Slavney PR. *The Perspectives of Psychiatry.* Second ed. Baltimore: Johns Hopkins University Press, 1998.

5. Costa PT, Jr., Widiger TA, eds. *Personality Disorders and the Five-Factor Model of Personality.* Second ed. Washington, D.C.: American Psychological Association, 2002.

6. Digman JM. Five robust trait dimensions: Development, stability, and utility. *J Pers* 57:195–214, 1989.

7. Goldberg LR. Some recent trends in personality assessment. *J Pers Assess* 36:547–560, 1972.

8. Hauser RM. Meritocracy, cognitive ability, and the sources of occupational success (CDE working paper no. 98-07). Madison: University of Wisconsin–Madison, Center of Demography and Ecology, 2002.

9. Neisser U, Boodoo G, Bouchard TJ, Boykin AW, Brody N, Ceci SJ. Intelligence: Knowns and unknowns. *American Psychologist* 51:77–101, 1996.

10. Frank JD, Frank JB. *Persuasion and Healing.* Third ed. Baltimore: Johns Hopkins University Press, 1991.

Chapter Two: The Psychiatric Evaluation

Epigraph. Bucknill JC, Tuke DH. *Manual of Psychological Medicine: Containing the History, Nosology, Description, Statistics, Pathology and Treatment of Insanity.* Philadelphia: Blanchard and Lea, 1858.

1. Kolb LC, Brodie HKH. *Modern Clinical Psychiatry.* Philadelphia: W. B. Saunders Company, 1934.

2. Slater E, Roth M. *Clinical Psychiatry.* London: Balliere, Tindall and Cassell, 1954.

3. Campbell WH, Rohrbaugh RM. *The Biopsychosocial Formulation Manual.* New York: Taylor and Francis Group, 2006.

4. Oyebode F. *Sims' Symptoms in the Mind.* Philadelphia: Elsevier, 2008.

5. Silverman K. *Edgar A. Poe: Mournful and Never-Ending Remembrance.* New York: HarperCollins, 1991.

6. Lyketsos CG, Chisolm MS. The trap of meaning: A public health tragedy. *JAMA* 302:432–433, 2009.

Chapter Three: The Life-Story Perspective

Epigraph. Jamison KR. *Nothing Was the Same.* New York: Alfred A. Knopf, 2009.

1. Folstein MF, Folstein SE, McHugh PR. "Mini-mental state." A practical method for grading the cognitive state of patients for the clinician. *J Psychiatr Res* 12:189–198, 1975.

2. Frank JD, Frank JB. *Persuasion and Healing.* Third ed. Baltimore: Johns Hopkins University Press, 1991.

3. Slavney PR, McHugh PR. *Psychiatric Polarities: Methodology and Practice.* Baltimore: Johns Hopkins University Press, 1987.

Chapter Four: The Dimensional Perspective

Epigraph. Osler W. On the educational value of the medical society. *Yale Medical Journal* 9:325, 1903.

1. Slavney PR. *Psychotherapy: An Introduction for Psychiatry Residents and Other Mental Health Trainees.* Baltimore: Johns Hopkins University Press, 2005.

2. Dekker MC, Koot HM, van der Ende J, Verhulst FC. Emotional and behavioral problems in children and adolescents with and without intellectual disability. *J Child Psychol Psychiatry* 43:1087–1098, 2002.

3. Costa PT, Jr., Widiger TA, eds. *Personality Disorders and the Five-Factor Model of Personality.* Second ed. Washington, D.C.: American Psychological Association, 2002.

Chapter Five: The Behavior Perspective

Epigraph. Sheff N. *Tweak (Growing Up on Methamphetamine).* New York: Atheneum Books, 2007.

1. Watson JB. *Behaviorism.* Revised ed. New York: W.W. Norton, 1930.

2. Pavlov IP. *Conditioned Reflexes as an Investigation of the Physiological Activity of the Cerebral Cortex.* London: Oxford University Press, 1927.

3. Skinner BF. *About Behaviorism.* New York: Alfred A. Knopf, 1974.

4. Bandura A. *Social Learning Theory.* Englewood Cliffs, N.J.: Prentice Hall, 1977.

5. Richter CP. *Biological Clocks in Medicine and Psychiatry.* Springfield, Il.: Charles C Thomas, 1965.

Chapter Six: The Disease Perspective

Epigraph. Rowling JK. *Harry Potter and the Deathly Hallows.* New York: Arthur A. Levine Books, 2007.

1. Rabins PV, Slavney PR. Overview of psychiatric symptoms and syndromes. In: Lyketsos CG, Rabins PV, Lipsey JR, Slaney PR, eds. *Psychiatric Aspects of Neurologic Diseases.* New York: Oxford University Press, 2008, p. 41.

2. Lage JM. 100 years of Alzheimer's Disease (1906–2006). *J Alzheimers Dis* 9:15–26, 2006.

3. Lerner DM, Rosenstein DL. Neuroimaging in delirium and related conditions. *Semin Clin Neuropsychiatry* 5:98–112, 2000.

4. Reischies FM, Neuhaus AH, Hansen ML, Mientus S, Mulert C, Gallinat J. Electrophysiological and neuropsychological analysis of a delirious state: The role of the anterior cingulate gyrus. *Psychiatry Res* 138:171–181, 2005.

5. Trzepacz PT. Update on the neuropathogenesis of delirium. *Dement Geriatr Cogn Disord* 10:330–334, 1999.

6. Brown AS, Derkits EJ. Prenatal infection and schizophrenia: A review of epidemiologic and translational studies. *Am J Psychiatry* 167:261–280, 2010.

7. Freedman R. Psychiatrists' role in the health of the pregnant mother and the risk for schizophrenia in her offspring. *Am J Psychiatry* 167:239–240, 2010.

8. Gilmore JH. Understanding what causes schizophrenia: A developmental perspective. *Am J Psychiatry* 167:8–10, 2010.

9. Maki P, Riekki T, Miettunen J, et al. Schizophrenia in the offspring of antenatally depressed mothers in the northern Finland 1966 birth cohort: Relationship to family history of psychosis. *Am J Psychiatry* 167:70–77, 2010.

10. Knopman DS, Roberts R. Vascular risk factors: Imaging and neuropathologic correlates. *J Alzheimers Dis* 20(3):699–709, 2010.

11. Demuro A, Parker I, Stutzmann GE. Calcium signaling and amyloid toxicity in Alzheimer Disease. *J Biol Chem* 285:12463–12468, 2010.

Case One: Bipolar Disorder

1. Beers C. A mind that found itself: A memoir of madness and recovery. Pittsburgh: University of Pittsburgh Press, 1908.

Case Two: A Young Man with Psychosis

1. Dragt S, Nieman DH, Becker HE, et al. Age of onset of cannabis use is associated with age of onset of high-risk symptoms for psychosis. *Can J Psychiatry* 55(3):165–171, 2010.

2. Gonzalez-Pinto A, Vega P, Ibanez B, et al. Impact of cannabis and other drugs on age at onset of psychosis. *J Clin Psychiatry* 69(8):1210–1216, 2008.

3. Rapoport JL, Addington AM, Frangou S, Psych MR. The neurodevelopmental model of schizophrenia: Update 2005. *Mol Psychiatry* 10(5):434–449, 2005.

Case Three: A Mother's Overdose

1. Costa PT, Jr., Widiger TA, eds. *Personality Disorders and the Five-Factor Model of Personality.* Second ed. Washington, D.C.: American Psychological Association, 2002.

2. Eysenck H. *Dimensions of Personality.* London: Kegan Paul, Trench, Trubner, 1947.

3. McHugh PR, Slavney PR. *The Perspectives of Psychiatry.* Second ed. Baltimore: Johns Hopkins University Press, 1998.

4. Littleton H, Axsom D, Grills-Taquechel AE. Longitudinal evaluation of the relationship between maladaptive trauma coping and distress: Examination following the mass shooting at Virginia Tech. *Anxiety Stress Coping,* 22:1–18, 2010.

5. Frank JD, Frank JB. *Persuasion and Healing.* Third ed. Baltimore: Johns Hopkins University Press, 1991.

Case Four: A Man with Depression amidst Multiple Life Stressors

1. Lyketsos CG, Chisolm MS. The trap of meaning: A public health tragedy. *JAMA* 302(4):432–433, 2009.

2. Wang PS, Berglund P, Olfson M, Pincus HA, Wells KB, Kessler RC. Failure and delay in initial treatment contact after first onset of mental disorders in the national comorbidity survey replication. *Arch Gen Psychiatry* 62(6):603–613, 2005.

3. Cuijpers P, Dekker J, Hollon SD, Andersson G. Adding psychotherapy to pharmacotherapy in the treatment of depressive disorders in adults: A meta-analysis. *J Clin Psychiatry* 70(9):1219–1229, 2009.

4. Brown GW, Harris TO, Kendrick T, et al. Antidepressants, social adversity and outcome of depression in general practice. *J Affect Disord* 121(3):239–46, 2009.

5. Post RM. Transduction of psychosocial stress into the neurobiology of recurrent affective disorder. *Am J Psychiatry* 149(8):999–1010, 1992.

Case Five: A Matriarch with Memory and Mood Problems

1. Rabins PV, Lyketsos CG, Steele C. *Practical Dementia Care.* New York: Oxford University Press, 2006.

Case Six: An Executive with Health Worries

1. Sakai R, Nestoriuc Y, Nolido NV, Barsky AJ. The prevalence of personality disorders in hypochondriasis. *J Clin Psychiatry* 71(1):41–47, 2010.

2. Kaminsky MJ, Slavney PR. Hysterical and obsessional features in patients with Briquet's Syndrome (somatization disorder). *Psychol Med* 13(1):111–120, 1983.

3. McHugh PR, Slavney PR. *The Perspectives of Psychiatry.* Second ed. Baltimore: Johns Hopkins University Press, 1998.

4. Slavney PR. The hypochondriacal patient and Murphy's "Law." *Gen Hosp Psychiatry* 9(4):302–303, 1987.

Case Seven: A Young Woman's Fear of Fat

1. Price JH, ed. *Modern Trends in Psychological Medicine.* Second ed. London: Butterworths, 1970, 131–164.

2. McHugh PR, Slavney PR. *The Perspectives of Psychiatry.* Second ed. Baltimore: Johns Hopkins University Press, 1998, 215–16.

Case Eight: A Lawyer Who Lies and Cuts

1. Paris J, Gunderson J, Weinberg I. The interface between borderline personality disorder and bipolar spectrum disorders. *Compr Psychiatry* 48(2):145–154, 2007.

2. Pope HG, Jr., Jonas JM, Hudson JI, Cohen BM, Gunderson JG. The validity of DSM-III borderline personality disorder. A phenomenologic, family history, treatment response, and long-term follow-up study. *Arch Gen Psychiatry* 40(1): 23–30, 1983.

Case Nine: A Case of Bereavement

1. Frances A. Good grief. *The New York Times*. August 15, 2010, Sunday Opinion, 9.

2. Slavney PR. Diagnosing demoralization in consultation psychiatry. *Psychosomatics* 40(4):325–329, 1999.

Index

abnormal perceptions, 27, 226
acquired activities, 10
addiction, 154, 235n2
agreeableness, 8, 113
Alzheimer, Alois, 65
Alzheimer disease, 7, 46
anorexia nervosa, 10, 176
anxiety, 45, 211; and behavioral disorders, 176; and depression, 141, 160
anxiety disorder(s), 141, 176
appearance, 113, 225
autism, 46

Bandura, Albert, 56
Beers, Clifford, 84
behavior, 55, 142; and appearance, 225; choice in, 9; disorders, 10, 11, 82, 97; extraordinary, 10; goal-directed, 55, 176; psychology's study of, 56; repetitive and acquired, 10, 82, 97; as something an individual does, 11, 55, 122
behavior perspective, 9–11, 54–55; in case histories, 50–54, 56–58, 82, 97, 116–17, 126–27, 140–41, 159, 175–76, 195–96, 209; treatment in, 11
biopsychosocial model, 3–4, 23
bipolar disorder, 82–83, 85, 176, 198
borderline personality disorder, 197–98
bulimia, 176

choice, 10, 54, 55, 126, 159; behavioral, 9
clinical syndrome, 7, 63–64, 65, 66

cognition, 8, 27, 45, 227
cognitive ability(-ies), 8, 141
collateral informants, 72, 80, 94, 110, 124, 137, 156, 173, 192, 207
comprehensive histories, 23–24, 161
conditioned learning, 10, 54, 126, 159
conditioning, 56
congestive heart failure (CHF), 63–64
conscientiousness, 8, 173
content of thought, 27, 227
Costa, P. T., Jr., 114

delirium, 65–66, 67
delusions, 27, 96, 160, 227
dementia, 5, 7, 64, 140–41
demoralization, 5, 11, 37, 96, 162
depression, 38, 160, 176; and dementia, 141–42; major, 46, 113, 128, 129, 142, 196–97
detailed history, 23
diabetes, 83, 97, 141
Diagnostic and Statistical Manual of Mental Disorders (DSM), 8–9, 117, 140; labeling focus of, x, 3, 23, 44; *Perspectives* approach and, 4, 215–16
diagnostic evaluation, 141–42
dimensional perspective, 8–9, 43–45; in case histories, 40–43, 81, 96, 113–16, 118, 125–26, 139–40, 158–59, 174–75, 194–95, 208–9; treatment in, 9, 48–49
disease perspective, 7, 63, 65; in case histories, 59–63, 64–67, 82–83, 97–98, 117, 127, 128, 140–42, 160–

www.ingramcontent.com/pod-product-compliance
Ingram Content Group UK Ltd.
Pitfield, Milton Keynes, MK11 3LW, UK
UKHW032035230425
457809UK00008B/284